Rising from the Flames

Rising from the Flames

The Experience of the Severely Burned

Albert Howard Carter III, PhD
and Jane Arbuckle Petro, MD

PENN

University of Pennsylvania Press

Philadelphia

id-free paper

Library of Congress Cataloging-in-Publication Data
Carter, Albert Howard, 1943–
    Rising from the flames : the experience of the severely burned /
Albert Howard Carter III and Jane Arbuckle Petro.
        p.   cm.
    Includes bibliographical references and index.
    ISBN 0-8122-3264-X (alk. paper)
    1. Burns and scalds — Psychological aspects.   2. Burns and scalds —
Social aspects.   3. Burns and scalds — Patients — Rehabilitation.
I. Petro, Jane A.   II. Title.
RD96.4.C375   1998
617.1′103 — dc21   97-46890
                                                                        CIP

Contents

List of Illustrations   vii

Acknowledgments   ix

A Note on Confidentiality   xi

Introduction: The Danger and Extremity of Severe Burns   1

Part I The Nature of Burns   9

1. What Are Burns?   11

2. Heat, Culture, and Betrayal   36

3. Burn Wounds — Damage by Accident or Intent   50

4. Prison or Nursery? Patients' Limitations in the Burn Unit   65

Part II Perceiving Burns Through Images and Stories   87

5. Myths of Fire and Burns   89

6. *Darkman* and Other Images of Burns in Popular Culture   105

7. Honey or Acid? A Short History of Burn Care   131

Part III Modern Care: Challenges to Patients, Families, and Caregivers   149

8. Contemporary Burn Care: "They Have All These Neat Things They Can Do Now"   151

9. Icarus Recovers (or Dies): How High Can a Survivor Fly?   177

10. Burn Care as a Stimulus for Medicine and Society   186

Epilogue   197

Appendix 1: Versions of the Phantom   201

Appendix 2: A Room Fire Illustrates Modern Fire Science   205

Bibliography/Filmography   207

Index   219

Illustrations

1a. Propane disaster   2
1b. Aerial view of propane tank in backyard   3
2. Lund-Browder chart   19
3. Skin cross-section, methods for determining burn severity.   21
4. "Medical prison"   66
5. Escharotomy   68
6a. Foot contracture   70
6b. Contracture treatment   71
7. Compression glove   72
8. Acute burn   76
9. Child's crib   77
10. Burn workers   78
11. Benu bird   103
12. "Napalm girl" by Huynh Cont ("Nick") Ut   106
13. Self-immolation for social protest, Saigon   107
14. Lon Chaney as Phantom of the Opera   112
15. Robert Englund as Freddy Krueger   114
16. Darkman as burn patient   116
17. Darkman, variation of the Phantom   117
18. Marshall Arisman, *Impact*   129
19. Cicatrices of face and neck   141
20. Electric dermatome   144
21. Skin mesher and knife   157
22. Legs covered by grafts   158

Acknowledgments

We gratefully acknowledge the help of many persons in making this book possible.

HC wishes to thank James F. Childress, leader of an NEH Summer Seminar on Metaphors and Principles in Biomedical Ethics at the University of Virginia. Also, the Center of Bioethics at the Kennedy Institute of Ethics for a year of study, particularly, LeRoy Walters, Warren T. Reich, Edmund D. Pellegrino, Laurence B. McCullough, and Marti Patchell. I am grateful to staff at four burn units where I have observed: Washington [D.C.] Hospital Center (Marion H. Jordan, M.D. and Cheryl J. Leman, O.T.R./L, M.A.) Grady Memorial Hospital, Atlanta (Roger Sherman, M.D.), Westchester [N.Y.] County Medical Center (see below), and, especially, Tampa General Hospital, where I observed over several years; I thank C. Wayne Cruse, M.D., Stephanie M. Daniels, B.S.N., Melinda A. Korte, C.L.P., Linda K. Attkisson, M.S., R.D., L.D., and many others there. I thank the staffs of the Emergency Room/Trauma Center and Pastoral Care (Mark Peterson, M.Div. in particular) at Bayfront Medical Center, St. Petersburg Fla., where I am a volunteer. I also thank Richard Selzer for early and important encouragement.

I further thank Lloyd W. Chapin, dean of faculty at Eckerd College, for research grants and leaves, also Molly K. Ransbury, Claire Stiles, and Thomas E. Bunch, successive chairs (during the writing of this book) of the Creative Arts Collegium. I also thank Robert Detweiler, director of the Dana Fellows Program at Emory University, of which I was a member during 1989–90, and Larry R. Churchill, chair, as well as Barry Saunders and W.D. White, Department of Social Medicine, University of North Carolina, Chapel Hill, where I was a visiting research professor during 1996–97.

I thank friends George and Karen Meese, Mary Ann Willis, Carolyn Horton, Susan Gill, and Mike Mader. I especially thank members of my family: Nancy (wife), Marjorie (mother), and Rebecca (daughter), who have given unfailing support.

JAP wishes to thank all of her patients. Their unique individual experiences have provided the source of continued professional growth and the stimulus for interest and enthusiasm for the practice of burn surgery which has lasted more than 25 years. Thanks also to student intern Heidi Taylor for her help in identifying and cataloguing comic book heroes, to Robert Arbuckle for his archival recovery of film stills and his recommendation of some of the films described in Chapter 6, and to Judy Carr-Collins for her contributions of materials related to the history of burn care, and the history of the American Burn Association. W. Bruce Fye of "Antiquarian Medical Books" in Marshfield, Wis., and Judith Miller of "An Uncommon Vision" in Wynnewood, Pa., helped locate out of print books and articles, and early burn texts and references. My partners in the Burn Center, Drs. Roger Salisbury and Andrew Salzberg, and the staff of the Burn Center at the Westchester County Medical Center, have my gratitude for the collegial atmosphere and intellectual climate which fostered the questions this book seeks to raise, and in part to answer. I also thank my family Carolyn and Noah for their patience and encouragement for this work.

We both thank the American Burn Association for its on-going work in burn research and burn care, also the Phoenix Society for Burn Survivors, Inc., for its work in care of burned patients and their families. We also thank the able staff of University of Pennsylvania Press, particularly Patricia Smith and Alison Anderson.

A Note on Confidentiality

We refer to many persons in this book, both patients and caregivers. We have taken due care to protect the confidentiality of both. Some cases, for example, have names and details changed; several are syntheses of parallel stories. Patients should be identifiable only in some cases already published in a newspaper article, say, or identified by a plaque displayed in a burn unit. An exception is the case of Tim (Chapter 8); we intend our use of his real name to serve as a tribute and a memorial to him.

Introduction: The Danger and Extremity of Severe Burns

A Propane Tanker Explodes

In July 1994 a tanker truck carrying propane fuel hit a bridge support in White Plains, New York. While the cab of the truck continued ahead, the propane tank exploded on impact, sending a massive fireball out one side and rocketing the tank back and to the other side (see Figure 1a). The fireball engulfed two buildings, a brick apartment house and a frame residence, and entered windows of the next house, igniting objects inside. In the more distant dwellings it caused small fires that were extinguished by the inhabitants, one of whom was the local fire chief. Residents of the brick building, however, were unable to fight the fires or use the fire escape, part of which was engulfed in flames. They fled to the roof, then lowered themselves by rope on the far side. Residents of the frame house also escaped but with serious burns. On the opposite side of the highway, the tank, still jetting burning fuel, crashed through the corner of one house and into the side of the next (Figure 1b). The most serious injuries to persons here were burns from radiant heat from the exploding propane and injuries sustained by leaping out of windows. A group of young men, playing cards at the time, leaped from the second floor of the house partly demolished by the passing tank. Residents more than a mile away were awakened by the sound and flash of the explosion. Twenty people required hospitalization for burns and related injuries. Four buildings were destroyed, twenty families made homeless, and a major interstate link closed for 23 hours.

The intense heat of the exploding propane and the different flammabilities of building materials produced a variety of burn injuries. Persons in the brick house had contact burns on their hands from the hot railing of the fire escape and on their feet from the tar roof of the burning house. Family members in the frame house sustained severe smoke and flame burns while escaping from the fire. Still others suffered flash burns as well as concus-

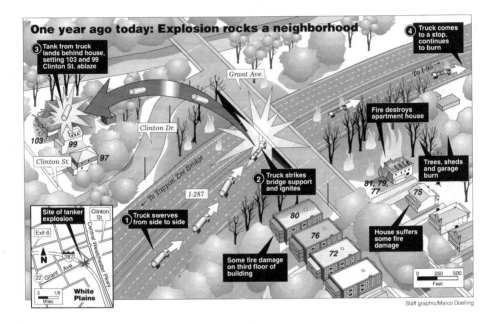

Figure 1a. A propane disaster. The diagram shows the events of the July 1994 White Plains, New York propane truck explosion. The numbers indicate locations where building damage occurred and generally coincide with sites of injury to people. Burn injuries ranged from severe to simple: flames produced severe burns on the legs and body of a two-year-old; heat produced sunburn-type burns on nearby residents. Graphic by Marco Doelling, Gannet Suburban Newspapers. Used by permission.

sions from jumping out of windows. Less serious were sunburn-type burns suffered by persons who stayed close to the flames while pouring water on their homes with garden hoses. Only the truck driver was killed, thrown from his cab.

Propane is one of the most volatile and flammable fuels available today. An efficient, clean-burning source of energy, it arrives at homes and businesses by truck, in liquid form under high pressure. Particular danger comes if the tank is subjected to sudden decompression, when a spark can detonate the leaking fuel. The gas dissipates rapidly, vaporizing into the air if no heat source ignites it, but when there is ignition disaster quickly follows. According to Arturson (1992), about 150 major disasters occur worldwide annually; of these, many are related to refined hydrocarbons, such as propane, and could occur only in modern times. In 1984 a disaster at a liquefied petroleum gas plant in San Juanico, Mexico killed 550 people and injured 7,000. In 1989 a train was engulfed by a natural gas explosion in Bashkir in the former Soviet Union, killing 530 and injuring 2,500. As in many disasters, the margin can be very small between "a close call" and

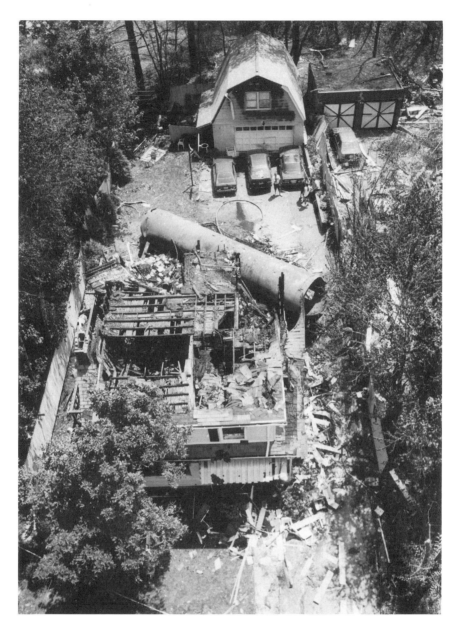

Figure 1b. Aerial view of the propane tank after it landed in a backyard. Photo by Stephen Schmitt, Gannett Suburban Newspapers. Used by permission.

complete chaos; the people in White Plains were unlucky that the propane ignited, but lucky that all the burns could be treated with modern medical care and no one died from them.

The various burns in the White Plains calamity called for different levels of care and yielded a wide range of final results, including post-traumatic stress syndrome (PTSS). Although everyone survived, almost no one seems to have resumed the same life as before the explosion. Members of family who fled the burning frame home suffered the worst injuries, including severe burns to the legs and body of a two-year-old carried out by the father. The parents had burns deep enough to require grafting. The mother was pregnant at the time. Labor was induced so that she delivered her baby 24 hours after the explosion, so that her burn care could go forward without harming the fetus. The baby, a girl, was born near-term and healthy; the birth — the first ever in the burn center caring for the family — provided a happy moment in the first hectic days following the disaster. The family eventually moved to a new home. They received counseling and social services support, gaining independence and readjusting relatively well. Their two-year-old, although severely injured, had survived; the new baby had been born safely. The parents had burn scars, but were functioning well. They received a large (and prompt) out-of-court settlement from the trucking and propane companies.

Other people had less dramatic injuries, but, paradoxically, some of these fared less well. Some of the injured, unable to work, lost their jobs. Burns to the hands and feet prevented others from prolonged standing, causing loss of work and school attendance. Finally, some patients did not keep any outpatient appointments, and how they fared is unknown.

This propane disaster introduces many of the topics and themes of this book. First, of course, is the dangerous and dramatic nature of burns themselves. Part I, "The Problematic Nature of Burns," discusses the difficulties posed by severe burns: the pain, the dilemmas in treatment, the many sources of heat (such as propane), the disruptions of meaningful life (accidents, warfare), and the many limitations that patients face, even those receiving modern care. The imperatives of biology and limitations of technology make serious burns terrible wounds for the patients who bear them and for the caregivers who must deal with myriad difficulties.

News media delight in showing pictures of fires because of their photogenic drama and primal appeal; an editor hearing of a large fire over the radio will often ask, "Is this worth aerial coverage?" The image of burns for humans is frightening, in part because of cultural and historical values based on many tragic meetings of fire and flesh. We discuss such values in Part II, "Perceiving Burns Through Images and Stories." Patients' assumptions based on these images, often out-of-date and misleading, may complicate their psychological state.

Part III, "Modern Burn Care: Challenges to Patients, Families, and Caregivers," explores how the modern medical response attempts to deal with the issues raised in the first two sections—both technical (grafts, prevention, rehabilitation) and social (counseling, healing the social imagination regarding burns). Modern burn units save thousands of patients a year who would have died at any time before, say, 1965. A typical mortality rate of a burn unit today in 3 percent; 97 percent leave the unit, often scarred and damaged, but alive, having survived an extreme event, a dangerous harm to body and mind.

Inquiring into Extremity

This book is about extremity, the outer limits of human experience in at least three senses, to use our discussion's organization just described: (1) the physical sense (heat out of control harms our flesh); (2) a traditional interpretive sense, the psychological and social meanings that give burns negative associations; and (3) the responsive sense, first, of the medical world that responds in ingenious and heroic ways and, second, of a wider humanistic context that sees and interprets the meaning and madness of burns to see their reality and their transformative power. Why should humans wish to examine such difficult and problematic topics?

There are many reasons why extremity fascinates human beings. Frontiers, whether geographical or intellectual, are calls to adventure, challenges: can we bring language and inquiry to deal with burns in depth? Can we look at stories, images, events from history and see how they shape, for better and for worse, our notions of burns? By their very nature humans like to explore the limits of the possible. Exploring extremity may even be an unavoidable obsession; it is innately human to do so. We can't help it; something deep within us compels us to know the limits of experience and expression. Our news media portray fires of all sorts: house fires, forest fires, industrial fires, and volcanic eruptions. We have a fascination with the chaotic reservoir of images of burns: hellfire, the fiery end of the world, nuclear holocaust, forms of torture, the fall of Icarus, the movie *Darkman* (1991), to name a few. Both psychologically and technologically, we are hooked on fire, but afraid of burns. This dual outlook suggests a cultural schizophrenia: the habitual use of fire as a highly controlled tool with the resultant estrangement from fire—real, present flames, alien to us and dangerous to our bodies and minds.

But of all the possible answers, the ones we like the best are the following. First, exploring extremity helps to situate ourselves somewhere within the bounds of normality; from this center, we have an increased sensitivity for the ranges of human experience and the need to care for those who encounter disaster, both patients and care-givers. Not all of us can or should work in burn units, but all of us meet people who hurt and can profit from any offered kindness. Thus our second claim for exploring extremity is this.

We mean to bear witness to persons who have been burned and to the persons who help those burned; there is a heroism in both groups of people that has passed unnoticed.

Although severe burns have the basic implied meanings of a dramatic event and subsequent pain, they do not, as a class of injuries, *mean* anything; that is, they do not—as wounds, as lesions—have any intelligible message or communication to make. Rather, interpretive meanings are *ascribed* to burns, by individuals, traditions, and cultures, which often allegorize burns directly into monstrosities or harbingers of death, *as if* burns had their own intentional, symbolic meaning. Some of the appeals of burns in popular culture assume the state of burn care of, say, a century ago, so that burn survivors are shown as monsters, scarred in body and mind. Such images influence the wider view of burns in a society, even when they are inaccurate and misleading.

An often-heard comment is "A burn is the worst thing that can happen to you." We've heard it in ordinary conversations, usually accompanied with a dismissive shrug or a shiver of disgust. We've even heard it from medical people: physicians, nurses, and technicians. One day some residents (young physicians, still in training) were talking about severe burns and one of them offered the "worst thing" formula.

Another doctor replied, "Yeah, it's a terrible injury all right, but is it any worse than a severe closed-head injury, break-bone fever, or end-stage AIDS? Besides, they have all these neat things they can do now for burns. They can bring back 90 percenters—to good lives!"

"Maybe so," another replied, "but I'll be damned if I'd ever want to have a severe burn," and others murmured their assent. Why do burns have such a dreadful reputation? Is it justified?

Severe burns are always and will always be with us, as long as humans work closely with heat and its powerful relatives. Nor will ignorance of burns or taboos against facing them help us; burns will not somehow "go away." Nor will varieties of blaming the victim help us; it is all too easy to say, "Well, he was careless; that burn should never have happened" as a way of hiding the fear of being burned ourselves and our vague hope that we will be so careful as never to have an accident.

Instead, then, we propose to tear away the veils of taboo, misinformation, and old-fashioned cultural images that surround and hide burns and to replace these with information, reinterpretation, and images and narratives that give us realistic but hopeful perspectives on burn. We will argue, for example, that the image of Icarus, falling from his high-tech flight toward the sun to his inexorable death in the sea, is symbolic of the fated and determined associations our culture has traditionally maintained about burns. This image is, however, misleading and outdated. The equally ancient story of the phoenix rising from its own ashes is in some ways more accurate and certainly more inspiring. Indeed the contemporary American burn survivor group calls itself the Phoenix Society for Burn Survivors, Inc. Founder and executive director Alan Jeffry Breslau speaks of the phoenix being reborn "more beautiful than before." Not all burn victims survive, of course: some plummet directly to death in spite of every technique of medicine, every effort on the caretakers' part, and many survive less beautiful in body and in mind. But many — and increasingly more — patients now survive and survive in better condition than ever before.

For the medical world, burns are a complex challenge, since every body system is involved. "If you want to learn medicine, do burns," is a common paraphrase of William Osler's aphorism, "Know syphilis in all its manifestations, and relations, and all things clinical will be added unto you" (1904, 140). The treatment of burns has a long and strange history, as humans have applied ingenuity and scientific methods to this field. There truly are "all these neat things they can do now" (see Chapter 8). Such medical treatment becomes part of the meanings of burns, especially for burn patients and their families who experience them first-hand.

Part I
The Nature of Burns

Chapter One
What Are Burns?

Burns are extreme events in the experience of humans; anarchic, painful, and nonlogical, burns are, to say the least, problematic. It is difficult to assign meaning to burns and to treat them medically, and yet humans have persisted in both areas. Attempts to define burns come from different perspectives, notably physical, cultural, and medical. After sketching these three areas, we will turn to definitions from specific groups of persons whose perspectives often vary greatly: patients, family and friends, and caregivers.

Physical Extremity

Although severe burn injury is at the margins of human experience, such burns usually happen in our common living and working areas. A disaster is always available — in any kitchen or bathroom, in the car or garage, in the workshop — anywhere there is a local, active, physical source of heat. The resultant injury touches on our skin, the dividing line between ourselves and the outer world. To destroy this protective membrane is to bring some element of the outer, physical world chaotically into our own personal physical world, our body habitus, to deconstruct our sense of outer and inner, even our sense of self-definition and identity. To burn flesh is to destroy it, either by killing the metabolic process of the cells, so that they slough, or by immediately vaporizing them into steam so that *part of us is utterly destroyed*. We all know the symbolism of burning a letter so that no one will see it again; to have part of our bodies similarly burned away *to nothing* is a horrifying concept. Even with lesser burns, there are many harms that can come to our flesh, and any harm to our life is, to our instinctive consciousness, extreme. While some burns are slow (exposure to the sun, for example), most happen very quickly, catching us off guard, sending us from good health to disaster in seconds. The intense physicality of burns — which will be implied by much of the following discussion — is perhaps the first and most basic quality that should be mentioned. (We will discuss the many biological harms of burns in Chapter 3.)

Traditional, Cultural Interpretations of Extremity

The burn event is usually a dramatic spectacle: a shower of sparks, a billowing fire, an exploding carburetor. Movie-makers, for example, love to show a stuntman aflame diving over the edge of a building. Why is this so? Certainly the spectacle is dramatic, an event at the edge of our experience, but perhaps the burning character also suggests a mythic scapegoat, a person we will, visually and hypothetically, push over the edge — so that we don't have to go there ourselves.

How should we deal with extremes and come to understand them? The easiest way, of course, is denial: to ignore them, hoping they will go away. This is the implicit strategy of our culture with many extreme topics. Thus we make them taboo, unspoken, undiscussed, uninquired. We do this with disability, disfigurement, and death itself. We certainly do it with burns. How often do we discuss burns in polite conversation? How often have any of us visited a burn unit? How often do we see a scarred survivor in public? Second, we tend to take the typical cultural definitions of burns as authoritative, so that figures from myth, literature, and popular culture become the unexamined norm. The devil, Frankenstein's monster, Freddy Krueger (the monster of the Elm Street films), and the main character in *Darkman* thus become our personifications for negative aspects of electricity, fire, and/or burns. Finally, burns bring forth our unexamined clichés and prejudices. Someone is severely burned; immediately we often assume that he or she did something wrong and somehow deserved it. We may imagine that he or she is going to be radically different because of this unspeakable experience, marked externally and internally. (We will return to such topics.)

Stephen Crane's short story "The Monster" (1899) serves as a good example of some of these associations. A black man is a hard-working groom for a doctor and his family. (Even his name, Henry Johnson, carries resonances of the folk hero John Henry.) When the doctor's house catches fire, Johnson runs in to save the young son. The fire, engulfing the doctor's laboratory, carries "all manner of odors," which "seem alive with envy, hatred, and malice" (Crane 1899, 205). The flames attacking are likened to a panther, a fairy lady, eagles, a "writhing serpent." It is the latter that does the most damage: "the red snake flowed directly down into Johnson's upturned face" (206). The newspaper announces Johnson's death, but the doctor saves him, scarred and a "monster." The townsfolk lament the doctor's effort, and say that Johnson should have died, that his brain is affected, that he scares normal people. One hand is a claw; he has no face; he is a devil. The word "monster" appears a dozen times or more. Unable to deal with mystery or abnormality, the town turns on the doctor, using gossip and social and economic shunning to make a scapegoat of the man who tried to help another man.

The story is told melodramatically, with lurid details. Like Mary Shelley's

Frankenstein (1818), it is ambiguous about who the monster is: the abnormal human, the scientist who produced him, or — most likely — the society that rages against extremity. In Crane's story, fire, disfigurement, and abnormality are more than the ordinary citizens are willing to deal with. They return, unthinking, to the small-town norms they know, cutting out of their society both the burn survivor and the physician who saved his life, as if ignorance were normal and proper. Here the extremes of the burn, both in the injury and in the treatment, are rejected, and both men become scapegoats for a society that cannot imaginatively embrace abnormality. This is a modern, much changed version of the story of Cain, the man who killed his brother and was cast out with his "mark of Cain" to wander the earth (Genesis 4). Although God's mark on Cain was originally meant to protect him from harm, it was later construed negatively, a sign of evil. Indeed Cain himself feared becoming a fugitive, a wanderer — an image kept alive in legends of the wandering Jew and, for the popular imagination, in persons scarred by burns. An external mark seems to ensure internal evil and to promote social isolation or shunning of this inferior person.

Can we heal our perceptions, our imaginations? As we look at some of the mythic, historical, and popular cultural images and stories that color our perceptions, we will critique these and attempt to disempower them. If we assume that there is social imagination regarding burns, can it be brought up to date or even healed from its morbid fascination with torturous pain, scars, and monsters?

Medical Responses to Extremity

Burn-care personnel have been hard at work in modern burn units for some thirty years, day in and day out, 24 hours a day, dealing with the extremities of burns. It is a hard profession, psychologically and physically. For example, burn units are usually kept quite warm to help conserve body heat in the immobile patients, and nurses and technicians ("techs") must move and lift patients for dressing changes, bathing, linen changes. Some caregivers transfer to a less demanding ward. Said one nurse, "I immediately gained ten pounds after leaving the unit."

The burn unit is a place that has evolved through much study, scientific research, and experimentation in burn treatments. While many people in medicine find other areas more congenial, interesting, or attractive, workers in the burn world have focused on burns as one of the ultimate challenges in medicine. Burn workers will typically say, "The unit is a tough place all right, but you can make so much difference in those people's lives!" Or even, "We're a different breed. You have to be ready to deal with a lot of really hard stuff in the burn unit."

Emergency workers are usually young, energetic, and eager to see extreme situations and to respond to them. Larry Brown, a retired firefighter, attributes much of the energy and heroic work of firefighters to adrenaline: "The adrenaline starts pumping when we run to the trucks. When the big starter kicks in and she rolls over and coughs like a dinosaur waking up, the adrenaline is flowing. It makes you not feel pain, not ignore it, actually, just *not even feel it* when it happens. . . . Adrenaline lets people do what they have to do, what they might not be able to do without it even if they had to" (Brown 1994, 5). Adrenaline is, of course, only one factor, but it helps explain why the burn unit attracts its workers and observers, whether doctors or nurses, writers or readers. The extremity of the wounds, the variety of the causes and patient attitudes, the closeness of life and death, the complexity of the medical dilemmas, and the surprises, both good and bad — all these are highly stimulating and challenging.

In many ways the burn unit is a world apart, a place that is not only intense and but also architecturally distant (by design — to avoid traffic and germs). Outsiders only learn about this world when they (or someone they know) are burned, they enter the unit, and they learn first-hand about the high-intensity care provided for burn patients. Burn-care personnel receive few of society's rewards, recognitions, or thanks, but families of burn patients know the expertise, the attention to detail, and the ability to face terrible wounds that characterize burn care; they also know the kind and encouraging words that typically accompany dressing changes, soaks, or physical therapy. By modeling how to deal with extremes, burn-care workers — physicians, nurses, techs, therapists, or others — give patients reassurance that they are not disgusting, hopeless, or entirely "ruined." Sometimes burn units have a wall of plaques proclaiming gratitude and thanks and even gifts of money for the unit; some of these praise the staff who returned a loved one to life, others are memorials for a patient who died in the unit. (See Epilogue for an example.) All is not always hearts and roses in the unit, of course, and many patients vent their anger at nurses, techs, physicians. One nurse matter-of-factly stated in rounds one day, "Mr. Freer screams so loud, and he won't leave his covers off to dry his wounds. But we'll work with him." Furthermore, many burn patients have suffered their wounds because of psychological turmoil, including alcoholism and drug abuse; they bring these dilemmas to the unit, where they must be treated along with the wounds. It also must be said that burn workers are as human as any other medical workers. They have feelings; they make mistakes. In a good burn unit there are enough support and quality control measures to minimize employee mistakes or other human failings. Blumenfeld and Schoeps emphasize this point in *Psychological Care of the Burn and Trauma Patient* with their final chapter "Care and Support of the Staff" (1993, 241–53).

Other exemplars of facing extremity are, of course, the patients and their friends and families. All these endure a crash course in burn care, suddenly dealing with the complexities of infection control, multi-system organ failure, uncertainties in the healing course, issues of life and death, and much more. It is a feeling of terrible helplessness to watch a loved one in intensive care, not knowing whether to be hopeful or to "prepare for the worst"; furthermore, such uncertainty may drag on for weeks. Often the burn staff cannot give any definite prediction because the patient's condition may change unexpectedly, and because severe burns are mysterious in affecting most or even all of the body's systems. A nurse might say, "Mrs. Franklin, in cases like this, usually they get better after some setbacks, but we never know exactly how it's going to go. Let's just take it a day at a time. Today, he's doing fine." Mrs. Franklin, of course, wants some words of certainty in the midst of the chaos that has taken her husband away from her. (See Munster et al. 1993, 30.)

Finally, the burn patients themselves are pioneers on these distant paths. Virtually none of them have chosen this role, not even the attempted suicides who put themselves aflame, but, willing or not, the profoundly burned person becomes our teacher about the limits of human physiology, psychology, and vitality. It is amazing to see a severely burned patient at intervals of, say, a week. The progress they can make is truly remarkable. This is not, however, to say that burn survivors live simply because of superior willpower; typically they are people much like the rest of us, and we too would "rise to the occasion" simply because we had no other choice. The healing capacity of the human body and mind, developed over millions of years, can, with the help of modern medicine, pull off amazing recoveries. We remember a burn nurse crying at a national burn meeting; she had learned that a particular unit gave only palliative care for the "90 percenters" (that is, gave up on healing them, assuming they would die). "What are they thinking of?" she wailed. "We bring most of these patients back, with quite acceptable results!" More accurately, her unit *and the innate capacities of the injured* brought the patient back.

Some Notes on Meanings

The meanings of burns come from many sources — medical, social, artistic, psychological. Thus there are different kinds of meanings, rational and irrational, up-to-date and out-of-date, social and cultural — all depending on the perspective of, say, a burn surgeon or a burn victim, a movie-goer or the spouse of a burned person. Indeed, the word "meaning" cannot be reductive in any sense, since burns are in some ways beyond language, primal entities that engage our sensibilities at deep and often inexpressible levels. In a search for meaning amidst chaos humans interpret burns as threat, as pain, as punishment, as damnation, as betrayal. This is an ancient urge to make sense of human mortality and tragedy; it is as old as the Babylonian *Epic of Gilgamesh* and the classic Greek plays. For example, by "treatments" we mean primarily medical treatments — a phrase that means Western-models of high-tech burn care. The wider, more metaphoric sense of "treatment," of course, blurs into work by artists, writers, the public at large, even each patient who must, day-by-day, week-by-week, make some sense of his or her burn.

Definitions of Burns from Various Points of View

Burns can be variously defined, depending on the person or tradition providing the definition: the definition given by a contemporary burn surgeon will differ from the definition of a "man on the street" or of a person who has survived a major burn. Definitions that imply kinds of treatment vary widely with their historical setting: a burn considered fatal in one decade may be readily treatable in another. All definitions face the difficulty, however, of bringing language to a phenomenon that is, in some ways, beyond language. Many burn survivors will say something like, "I don't remember a lot of the time in the unit, but what I do remember is impossible to put into words." We appreciate this dilemma, in its various psychological, linguistic, and philosophical dimensions: in some ways burns are truly ineffable, beyond the range of definition by words.

Nonetheless, humans have struggled with many concepts on the edge of our verbal abilities, burns included. Furthermore, our senses of adventure, pioneering, and reckoning with the unreckonable seem to draw us into bringing language and systematic thought to bear on this troublesome entity, burns. It must also be said that modern medical definitions — however limited they are in some dimensions — are remarkably effective in making possible excellent burn care. In this chapter we will discuss various definitions of burns: medical definitions; personal definitions of burn survivors, their family, and friends; definitions of burn-care works; and, finally, some of the pervasive metaphoric and psychological meanings.

Medical Definitions

The medical definitions are the rational, denotative formulas we might expect of a scientific and academic discipline. Here are three examples: "the tissue reaction or injury resulting from application of heat, extreme cold, caustics, radiation, friction, or electricity" (*Blakiston's Gould Medical Dictionary*, 1979); "injury to tissues caused by contact with dry heat (fire), moist heat (steam or hot liquid), chemicals (e.g., corrosive substances), electricity (current or lightning), friction, or radiant and electromagnetic energy" (*Dorland's Illustrated Medical Dictionary*, 1988); and "lesion caused by heat or any cauterizing agent, including friction, electricity, and electromagnetic energy" (*Stedman's Medical Dictionary*, 1990). These definitions then go on to describe the classification system of first-, second-, and third-degree burns (which we will discuss in a moment).

Each of these definitions has two components. First is the concept of *injury* or *damage* to human flesh, specifically the burned area of tissue, which will be the focus of this chapter. We use various words — wound, lesion, injury — more or less interchangeably, although each has different connotations. "Wound" may suggest violent action, as in war wounds. "Lesion" is a more strictly medical term, meaning damage to tissue by injury or disease. ("Lesion" has a cousin in the phrase "lèse majesté," a crime against a ruler or sovereign, in short, treason; perhaps we feel that the majesty of the human body has been betrayed by a burn.) "Injury" carries a hidden meaning in its Latin root "injurius," or "unjust."

But these definitions from medical dictionaries offer no hint of pain, which is central to the experience of burns. (*Stedman's* gives another sense: "to suffer pain caused by excessive heat or similar pain from any cause" as in the burning feet of a diabetic, but pain is not part of the definition of a thermal injury.) These three medical definitions are technical, not experiential or personal. Clearly we are in a realm of perception that seeks to be objective, not subjective, neither personal nor social. We are also in a realm of tight focus, so that the injury is local, distinct, a specific "tissue reaction." None of these definitions mentions secondary but very important effects such as burn shock (historically, one of the biggest killers of patients with major burns), burn infection (now one of the major causes of death), damage to other body systems, or changed metabolic status of the patient (who will need more calories than usual). And there are the further associational, connotative meanings that patients and their families have, meanings which guide their interpretation and response to the burn and its aftermath.

We argue here that the strict medical definition is a kind of linguistic objectification and limitation typical of the scientific view, and that there are advantages to this style of denotative definition, such as clarity, tight focus, clinical distancing, and even self-protection of caregivers. But there are also profound disadvantages, such as loss of humanity of patients, their whole-person dignity, their attempts — even desperate attempts — to make sense of their calamities, and the need for a "full-spectrum" dialogue that will become part of the healing. A further issue is the risk of self-delusion: that medical language attempts rational control through reductionism. While there are some advantages to medical objectivity, a disadvantage can be a tight focus of perception that overlooks other injuries, such as fractures or a damaged spleen — especially from high-energy trauma — while aggressively treating the clearly evident burns.

The second aspect evident in the three medical definitions is the *agent* of the burn: heat, chemicals, radiation, even friction. We have no fundamental quarrel with these; we discuss them in Chapter 2. We might add only that burn units sometimes treat patients with skin that breaks down for other reasons: frostbite, Stevens-Johnson syndrome (in which the patient sloughs skin, typically as a drug reaction) or toxic epidermal necrosis syndrome (TENS), and some genetic illnesses, such as epidermolysis bullosa, or acquired disorders such as pemphigus. All these cause injuries to patients that are similar to burns and are, therefore, treated like burns.

Burns are injuries to the skin, the largest organ of the body by weight and one of the most crucial to our health and well being. Burns start from the outside and work their way in, whether the agent is heat, chemicals, or radiation. Even electrical energy starts from the outside, although its most serious damage may not be on the surface: current may choose nerves, arteries, or other deep structures, such as bone and muscle, as conduits toward ground. With the exception of some electrical injuries, burns are highly visible to everyone, the victim included. The first medical descriptor of a burn, then, is the amount or *area* of the body damaged, expressed in percentage of total body surface area (TBSA).

The standard method for estimating the percentage of skin burned is the Lund-Browder chart (see Figure 2), which follows a modification of the Rule of Nines, by which body sections were calculated as equal to 9 percent of the TBSA. (There are variations for children, whose proportions are different.) Physicians will draw on this schematic analogue, adding up body sections to reach a total number. The higher the number, the more serious the injury and the more aggressive the treatment required.

Surface is not the only dimension, of course, since depth — the second descriptor — is crucial too. Thus physicians will mark on the Lund-Browder chart estimates of depth of the burn, so the final description may be "a 60% TBSA burn with 40% full thickness." This number may prove inaccurate, since burns can be deceptive in their appearance and can evolve (or "convert") from a superficial to a deeper wound over the next twenty-four hours, but it is a good place to start with treatment.

There are two modern systems for depth assessment. The older one (which has roots in Dupuytren's classification of six levels) gives three or four levels of burn injury, or "degrees." (For a full discussion of classifications going back to 1607, see Harkins 1942, 18–21.) *First degree* means that the outer layer of skin, the epidermis, is reddened. A mild sunburn is a good example, as are minor burns from water, hot pots, or fires. There may be swelling, but no blisters. *Second degree* means that the epidermis and the next layer, the dermis, are damaged. Usually there are blisters, which may be superficial or deep. Some may burst, releasing fluid from the body and leaving the body open to infection. (Some second-degree burns can heal themselves, some cannot; hence the alternate classification system.) *Third degree* means that heat has seriously damaged the dermis, so that the skin is destroyed all the way through. Some authorities suggest a fourth degree, damage to underlying muscle or even bone.

Contemporary care, however, has switched to different terminology for describing depth. This classification provides operational definitions: how

Westchester County Medical Center
Burn Center
Lund Browder Chart

Westchester County Medical Center

ADDRESSOGRAPH:

Area	Birth-1 yr	1-4 yr	5-9 yr	10-14 yr	15 yr	Adult	Partial	Full
Head	19	17	13	11	9	7		
Neck	2	2	2	2	2	2		
Anterior trunk	13	13	13	13	13	13		
Posterior trunk	13	13	13	13	13	13		
Right Buttock	2½	2½	2½	2½	2½	2½		
Left buttock	2½	2½	2½	2½	2½	2½		
Genitalia	1	1	1	1	1	1		
Right upper arm	4	4	4	4	4	4		
Left upper arm	4	4	4	4	4	4		
Right lower arm	3	3	3	3	3	3		
Left lower arm	3	3	3	3	3	3		
Right hand	2½	2½	2½	2½	2½	2½		
Left hand	2½	2½	2½	2½	2½	2½		
Right thigh	5½	6½	8	8½	9	9½		
Left thigh	5½	6½	8	8½	9	9½		
Right leg	5	5	5½	6	6½	7		
Left leg	5	5	5½	6	6½	7		
Right foot	3½	3½	3½	3½	3½	3½		
Left foot	3½	3½	3½	3½	3½	3½		
						Total		

Age: _____

Sex: _____

Weight: _____

24 Hour Fluid **ESTIMATE:** _____

Hour 0-8 _____ cc/hr

Hour 9-24 _____ cc/hr

Pediatric Maintenance: _____ cc/hr

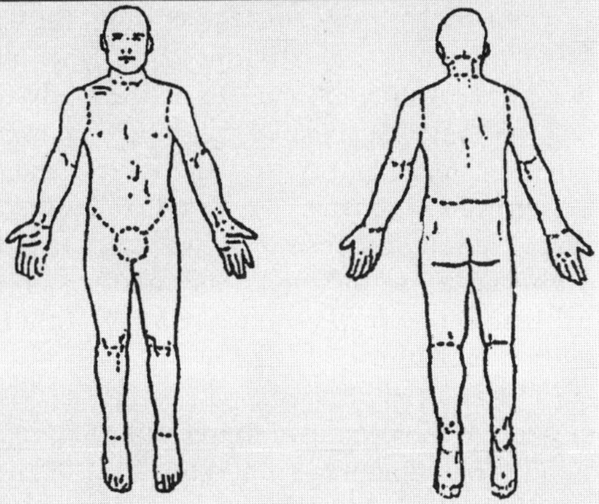

HC-482-93

Figure 2. Lund-Browder chart. This is a typical form used to designate areas and severity of burn injury when patients are admitted to a burn center. On the body outline (lower right) red is used for areas of full thickness injury (third degree) and blue for partial thickness (second degree). The chart as originally designed used the Rule of Nines, ascribing 9 percent each to the arms and head, 18 percent to the front and back of the trunk, and 18 percent to each whole leg. This newer version permits a more precise estimate of the extent of injury, allowing calculations when whole parts are not involved. These estimates are valuable in planning both patient resuscitation and subsequent fluid and caloric requirements.

the burns will behave over time and what treatments are, therefore, the most appropriate for each level (see Figure 3, showing both terminologies). Starting again with the least serious burns, we have *superficial* burns, which damage only the epidermis. The next level is *partial thickness*, which means that the dermis is damaged but the wounds can heal on their own in about three weeks; there is enough skin, particularly down in hair follicles, to grow up and out, meeting across the wound bed. Next comes the *deep partial*, which means the dermis is more deeply affected, and that it would take more than three weeks for regrowth; thus grafting new skin over the burn early in treatment makes sense. Finally, we have *full thickness* burns, which means that tissue is badly damaged or killed all the way through the two major layers of skin. Such a burn will not heal without a graft.

What is the actual damage? In the most extreme case, total destruction, the skin cells superheat, their liquid contents boil, and the cell walls explode. Less dramatic, but equally deadly, is disruption of all metabolic activities of the cell, so that the cell dies. If the cell's protein coagulates, it turns white and opaque, much as egg white or a fillet of fish changes color in a frying pan. (Large numbers of dead and dehydrated cells can create an eschar, a crust of dead tissue, usually dark and leathery; this is dangerous, a nursery for bacteria, and must be removed.) The next lower level of intensity is sufficient injury to the cell to kill it later, even several hours later. Such irreversible injury may occur because insufficient oxygen has reached burned tissues. Next we have damaged tissues which may or may not return to health, depending, for example, on adequate fluid resuscitation and oxygen delivery. Finally we have cells that have been heated but not beyond the capacity of the body to recover; these cells will appear reddened (particularly in lightly pigmented people), as in a sunburn, when increased blood flow attempts to heal damage. (While we have mentioned mild sunburn as a typical first-degree or superficial burn, it is important to mention that serious sunburn can cause a second-degree burn and even lead to death when combined with factors, such as heat stroke, dehydration, or sun poisoning — to say nothing of skin cancer that appears twenty years later.)

Cells, in brief, are sacks of protein, saltwater, and nucleic acid, all contained in a membrane of lipids. They live at around 98.6° F (37° C) and can stand slightly higher temperatures. At about 110° F (42° C), however, the protein starts to denature (technically the molecules uncoil; figuratively, the very nature of life is coming apart). Denaturing is sometimes reversible; actual coagulation (above 113° F (45° C)) is not. At that point cellular death is guaranteed.

Many serious burns have all these levels of injury, often as concentric circles around the most severe burn, at the point of thermal contact. There are, of course, further medical aspects to burns, many of which will be discussed in Chapter 3.

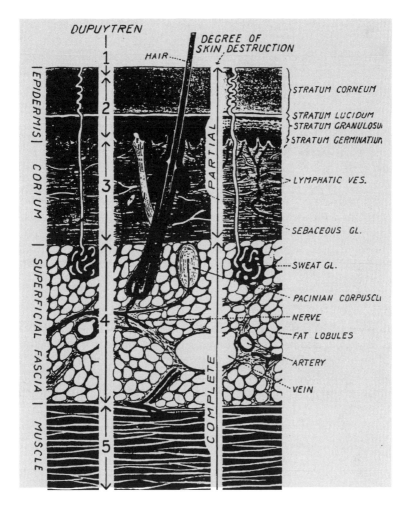

Figure 3. Skin cross-section showing two methods for determining burn severity. The classification used by Dupuytren, dividing the levels of burn injury into six categories, has been superseded by the description of skin injuries in terms of partial and full thickness. These labels help predict healing based on the amount of viable skin elements preserved in the burn wound and guide plans for surgical intervention.

Burns According to Patients

A burn may be defined as a specific injury to tissues, but it also has a profound effect on the mind of the patient. The initial burn event is usually dramatic and horrifying, and the healing course, with many difficult treatments, is grueling, demeaning, and lengthy (none of these adjectives are, of course, adequate).

Books by (or about) burn survivors detail the intensity of their experiences of mind and body. Mary Ellen Ton reports rage at seeing her face for the first time after her burn (Ton 1982, 63). She also says that pain was so bad that "Death became very alluring — quite beautiful, in fact, when seen as an escape from pain" (40); on arriving home, she feels she is a monster (84, 95). David Snitker reports that the pain was "pure hell." "It was everywhere, and it was nowhere, I couldn't grab hold of it, or run away from it, or stop it — even for an instant. There are no words to explain the way it sucked my strength, and drained my mind as I worked constantly to hold myself and my mind together" (Snitker 1983, 24–25). Snitker also sees his wounded body as a monster. Diane Bringgold found her burns to be the occasion of pain, loneliness, and grief (Bringgold 1979, 24). Her husband and three children were killed in the plane crash that severely burned her; she writes, "Sometimes in the middle of the night I did let the tears flow. 'Why me, Lord?' I would cry. 'Why did you take my wonderful family?' " (50). Later, she can do errands in town, wearing her compression garments; a child asks her if she is a monster — and she is able to joke about it (89). Sometimes survivors emphasize the reactions of others, who perceive them as monsters (Rothenberg and White 1985, 203). Alan Jeffry Breslau assesses his wounds with an engineer's eye and intelligence, often using medical language, but he also reports extensive pain and nightmares (Breslau 1977). He concludes that looks or handicaps are not in themselves important, rather it is his spirit and resolve and that of his friends. His wounds became technical absurdities that he could overlook and overcome through social contacts (phoning his family, for example) and self-hypnosis (168, 182).

In each of these cases, personal attitude was an important factor in the healing of the wounds. For Ton, Snitker, and Bringgold, the faith was religious, specifically Christian. Breslau, who is Jewish, saw his wife's faith as crucial, although it was "not a religious faith" (164); he also felt that his own resolve was crucial: "I wasn't fighting to live; I just never conceived of dying" (170). The burns were many things to these writers, but several qualities stand out: the pain, the self-questioning, the monstrous appearance, the anger and despair, as well as the inner resources that somehow developed and held firm through the long ordeal. Much of the rest of this book will elaborate on the need for comprehensive treatment of any patient — body, mind, and soul (see Chapter 9).

A patient arriving at a burn unit for treatment will have little understanding of the medical definitions of percentage and depth. The patient's understanding will not even be on a definitional or categorizing level; indeed even the concept of meaning itself may have little bearing. The patient with a serious burn will likely be in shock, dulled by pain-relieving drugs, perhaps entirely unconscious. The many levels of meaning and implications of burns will emerge over the next several weeks, and most of these will be metaphoric, not technical. *What is the image of this burn for me? How will this burn affect my life? Will my spouse still find me attractive? Will I be scarred? Will people laugh at my stupidity? Will I be a monster? Will I have anything like a normal life ever again?* Such profound questions pivot on the associational and often half-conscious definitions of burns in the past experience of patients as well as their sudden — and often desperate — need to create meanings to explain their tragedies.

An excellent discussion of images of body disfigurement is a memoir by Lucy Grealy, "Mirrorings: To Gaze upon My Reconstructed Face" (1993). Grealy describes a twenty-year ordeal with facial cancer and the punishing treatments of surgery and chemotherapy that caused her much physical and psychological pain. (Most of the burn patients we've talked to also mention pain immediately as part of their burn experience.) The psychological difficulties with her disfigured face caused her to lead an introverted life; she views herself as a reject of society, someone who is teased and stared at by children. Eventually she sees her physical state as a symbol for her mental state: "I became unable to say 'I'm depressed' but could say only 'I'm ugly,' because the two had become inextricably linked in my mind" (73). (This linking of physical image and mental state is similar to the social perception of the monster in Crane's short story: *he looks bad; he must be bad.*) After thirty reconstructive operations, Grealy's notion of her identity was confused: "It wasn't only that I continued to feel ugly; I simply could not conceive of the image as belonging to me. My own image was the image of a stranger, and rather than try to understand this, I simply stopped looking in the mirror" (74). Grealy writes that intellectually she understood that the image of her face was just a surface, but experience in society led her to conclude: "that our whole lives are dominated . . . by the question 'How do I look?'" (74). She concludes, "it is our own sense of how we appear to the world by which we chart our lives, how we navigate our personalities, which would otherwise be adrift in the ocean of *other* people's obsessions." Rejecting social pressures and definitions, she seeks to recognize herself in her reflection not only in a mirror, but also in her thinking and feeling — in short, in her reflective mind.

This moving and illuminating essay makes clear the profound links we have between our physical looks, how others see us, and how we see ourselves. The word "image" has an appropriate ambiguity: the first sense is of the object directly perceived visually, but the second sense is of the attributed metaphoric meanings that cluster around, in this case, her face. When she stops allowing others to make the interpretations and takes responsibility for her own direct vision of herself and the interpretation of what she sees, the essay can conclude on a triumphant and hopeful note. This essay won a 1994 National Magazine Award and has since been expanded to a book (*Autobiography of a Face*, 1994).

Another word with a dual meaning is "insult." In medical circles it means the harm suffered by the body because of an outside force, such as a bullet or boiling water. In common usage it means, of course, words or actions that are disrespectful or even contemptuous. (The Latin roots for both meanings are instructive: something *leaps onto* us.) Combining both meanings of insult for burns yields a definition like this: *an evil or malevolent force that has ambushed us unfairly, creating a bad image that will cause other people to look down on us.* A burned or otherwise maimed person often feels both meanings of the insult, the outside attack and the psychological loss, which may be perceived from the condescending views of others. The word "image" is, of course, the basis for the word "imagination," that creative and interpretive power of the mind. The individual imagination of each patient is important as a resource for motivation in healing; indeed there have even been speculations that an engaged imagination can influence the healing course, for example through the immune system. Imagination can definitely influence the patient's contributions to healing, as he or she can envision the future, for example — images that may influence cooperation in physical therapy, wearing compression garments, and eating enough calories to grow new skin.

Grealy's experience and articulate interpretation can be applied directly to the world of burns. If they look in a mirror, most patients feel profound discomfort with the dramatic change of their looks — in the primary burn wounds, in the secondary wounds of graft sites, in the copious bandages, in the loss of movement and physical grace, even in the fright in their eyes. Most burn units have no mirrors available at random on walls, where patients could see them from their beds. Rather — if present at all — mirrors are commonly over bathroom sinks: patients must be well enough to walk that far to use such mirrors. Alternatively, staff may give patients a hand-mirror when they seem ready to confront how they look.

Gretel Ehrlich, a poet, writes about being struck by lightning in her *A Match to the Heart* (1994). She reports that she suffered burns shaped like ferns (so-called arborescent erythema) over her body, paralysis (temporary except for her more severely damaged right arm), a concussion, broken ribs, a possible broken jaw, and lacerations. Her recovery is slow because of cardiac and neurological problems caused by the passage of electricity through her body. For her, it is not strength of will or faith that brings her back, but a mysterious process, during which she feels like an exile (66), in a "wide-awake coma" (72). She studies nature, writings, the possible meanings of her life. She seems to gain strength and support from the Third

Annual Lightning Strike and Electric Shock Conference. There she learns of other strange journeys somehow parallel to hers, and she embraces life once again.

Part of the recovery of burn patients, then, is the rebuilding of a psychological image about themselves as well as healing the specific tissues burned.

Some patient definitions are surprising, even delightful.

> One day during rounds an elderly woman suddenly asked one of the resident physicians, "Have you ever been to the moon?" He was taken aback and began to wonder whether this patient would need psychiatric help; nonetheless he said, "No, I haven't." The woman continued, "Well, you won't have to. Have a look at this" and held out her unbandaged arm, burned, grafted, and scarred. "Looks just like the moon, doesn't it, with craters, gullies—all sorts of strange things!"

For her, the arm was a wonder, a miracle of survival, perhaps even on an astronomic or cosmic scale. For the resident, it was "a deep partial burn with an 80 percent take of a split-thickness graft." Might his technical definition start to share space in his mind with her lunar image?

For the patient, a burn is also an event in continuing time. It has been said frequently that *a severe burn lasts forever*, even if the patient is considered healed by ordinary standards. The dramatic events of the burn, the protracted treatments, the resulting physical limitations, and psychological residue typically stay with a patient for a very long time. A burned person wears the mark of the event, both externally (even if only he or she can discern it) and internally. If the event was an accident, the patient may feel that the world is unjust and absurd. If the event was intentional, the patient may feel that betrayal and hatred infuse all reality. If the burn was a failed suicide attempt, the patient may feel disappointment, or shame, or joy. As people and burns vary widely, so do the psychological impacts, but it is probably safe to say that for all patients such impacts are strong and protracted. Severe burns, then, are life-changing events. Each patient leaves a particular routine of life with a dramatic event and enters the new world of the burn unit with its rules, traditions, and treatments, then slowly reenters the public world. (This re-entry is often problematic; see Chapter 9.)

The process is in many ways a regression to early childhood followed by a re-birth: in the acute stage of the burn the patient returns to a state much like infancy, being fed and changed, slowly sitting up, standing up, taking first steps — all under the care (or domination) of "parents." (For patients who die, the regression also occurs, but not the rebirth.) Many patients rebel against this process, much as adolescents rebel against authority. Oliver Sacks writes about the routine rebelliousness of recovering trauma patients, himself included, in his book *A Leg to Stand on* (Sacks 1984, 166–67). William F. May finds religious implications in the sequence "life/death/rebirth" (1991, 20–28). Some patients create their own rituals to celebrate the anniversary of their burns or their release from the hospital, a second birthday, in effect. (We'll return to this in Chapter 4.)

We see from the preceding paragraphs that attempts to define burns may easily spread to wider concepts. In English, the word "burn" is both a noun (an occurrence) and a verb (an action). A burn happens as an event in time, and also an action, a dynamic blow inflicted by the world upon a person: a man may have poured lighter fluid on a barbecue fire many times without incident, but suddenly he finds his arm and torso engulfed in flames. The burn, for him, is many things: pain, betrayal, loss of order, frightful surprise, and an entry into weeks of burn treatment. The healing (or dying) may stretch on for weeks and months, and after-effects will be with him for life. For patients, the time in the hospital (often six weeks) is a time to reflect on life, personal goals, relationships, values, and priorities. Some patients make pivotal decisions for their lives. Occasionally one will say, "You know, in a funny kind of way it was a good thing that I got burned — not that I'd ever do it again. But I've had the time to look over my life, which really wasn't going anywhere, and set myself some new directions." For such a patient, the burn may be defined as rebirth, transformation, or passing through the refiner's fire. Some patients are able to escape alcohol and/or drug addictions because of detoxification begun during burn treatment.

For others, however, the burn is just one more event in a sad parade. Many burn patients come from the margins of society: poor people, street people, "bums." A very common event is this: incapacitated by liquor and/or drugs, a homeless person falls into his or her campfire. Paramedics bring such burned street people to the unit, where their healing course is often slow because of their generally poor health, suppressed immune systems, and the like. On leaving the hospital (if they survive), they typically return to the same life, perhaps even another life-threatening accident. They rarely come to a clinic for follow-up, and there is no specific social agency caring for their rehabilitation. (In a mood of exasperation — and realism — a physician wrote a discharge order for a patient living at "the second bush from the end of Pelston Ave. and Wingate St." Visiting nurses actually made their calls to that location.) Indeed, it is only recently that Social Security has acknowledged that burns cause disability that may qualify for aid. A second severe burn for such patients will usually end their lives, although some survive, often to the amazement of burn unit personnel. Sadly enough, the rate of burns among this population is disproportionately high, as if our society were content, somehow, to burn these people up.

A more unusual definition of burns is this. For a disturbed person a burn is a dramatic and climactic way of concretizing psychological turmoil. Disappointed lovers sometimes burn themselves — or their lovers, or their children — to show the other person how deeply they have been hurt. Sometimes this is described as "acting out," a phrase that may provide some truth or insight, in that the physical action portrays inner dynamics. But surely more is involved here, since the burn event may also be, for the person lighting the match, a promise of justice or relief. In a strange kind of way, therefore, the burn is a coping mechanism. If the patient survives, the protracted hospital stay will be a time for not only reflection but psychiatric attention: ironically, the burn brings treatment that is unforeseen but deeply needed. The spurned lover may persist in the interpretation that the burn was a lesson to the former lover, but, as he or she recovers, the burn will take on other meanings as well.

Burns may mean many things for patients. Perhaps the most fortunate patients are those whose sense of a burn can evolve from tragedy to a deeper understanding of positive change in the vulnerable but miraculous lives of humans.

Burns According to Family and Friends

There is much variety in these perspectives as well, since people come from all areas of life, but most of them know very little of the trauma world in general or the burn world in particular. Entering the world of intensive care, infection control, and high-tech medicine may be like a visit to another planet. Even putting on a mask can be a challenge: an unusual action, perhaps associated with criminals, and an oppressive structure that changes sensations of breathing. Re-breathing carbon dioxide can cause dizziness. All these factors combined may cause a first-time visitor to faint, as Alan Jeffry Breslau reports (162).

Many people are afraid of hospitals, for the usual reasons: they fear death, they fear the unknown, they fear the lack of control for the patient and for themselves. But these same people are especially important for burn patients, as they provide a continuity to the outside, continuing world. Furthermore, such people are educable in the sense that orientation to the burn unit and practice through short visits can make it less foreign and threatening. Except for psychotic or highly introverted survivors, all burn patients report that the support of outsiders is a big factor in shaping their own attitudes toward survival, rehabilitation, eating, and the like. One man thanked his fellow workers who brought (or sent) cards, flowers, banners, posters, books, and balloons making sure that something cheery and colorful would arrive everyday. "I wanted to make it to the next day just to see what they'd come up with next," he said. The creative meanings his friends attached to his burn helped him to redefine his experience as well: "I never knew so many people cared that much about me," he said in wonder.

We will return to the role of "outsiders" in Chapter 9, where we will argue that they may be best understood as part of the burn team. One progressive burn unit has a carefully designed waiting room for the visitors' lounge, with cheerful decorations and plenty of information about burns and burn care.

Burns According to Caregivers

Earlier we reviewed some of the technical meanings of burns from medical dictionaries. While these are formative of caregivers' attitudes, they are not absolute: burn workers are also aware of their patients' suffering, and it's safe to say that they have all suffered minor burns themselves and that many have suffered significant personal injury or illness. (Indeed, many health workers enter the field because of their experiences of healing, either of themselves or of close family members.) We are also aware of the diversity of perceptions and interpretations among burn-care personnel, so we make no claims that all workers would subscribe to all ideas below. We have, however, heard these ideas from many people, so we know that many of them are common.

One of the most common views is that burns are an opportunity to help. We have asked many people why they work in the burn unit — one of the hardest jobs in a hospital — and they will often reply, "You can make such a difference in people's lives." The wounds are severe, but the progress, week by week, is clear. Because units are small — often ten to twenty beds — and the nursing ratios are low (one-to-one in intensive care, one-to-three or -four in the step-down unit), nurses and other staff get to know patients and their families quite well over, say, four weeks. There is deep satisfaction in the healing of a person who arrives in terrible shape but who can walk out the door — unassisted — some weeks later.

Burns are also a wily opponent, complicated, evolving, a persistent challenge to skills, strategies, and technologies. Burn workers take pride in working with such difficult injuries. "We're a different breed" is a phrase we have often heard. They seem to enjoy bringing their collective thinking to focus on some of the most brutal and complicated injuries in the hospital. At a recent burn conference a nurse-practitioner said: "We tell our new nurses that the burn unit will allow them to use everything they learned in nursing school." A plastic surgeon nodded in agreement: "And I tell surgery residents 'if you want to learn surgical illness in depth, do a lot of burns.' "

Burn rounds bring together representatives of seven or so different professional perspectives: physician, nurse, nutritionist, physical therapist, occupational therapist, psychiatrist, social workers, and perhaps others, such as a chaplain. Some units may have twenty people present at rounds, including interns and medical students. Rounds therefore are a chance to fit different pieces of the puzzle together, from the nature of the original injury to on-going concerns of the different disciplines concerning infections, splinting, exercise, mental attitude, and later, rehabilitation, out-placement, and aftercare. The professional organization for burns in the United States is the American Burn Association, which prides itself on the diversity of its membership across various medical professions.

Burns are also a kind of an abyss to peer into, a brush with death, a facing of extremity. For some workers, it is a way of testing yourself, seeing what you are made of, putting you "on your mettle." A negative side of this can be the kind of thrill-seeking or search-for-adrenaline response Larry Brown mentions, but these are not sufficient to maintain long-term service in a burn unit; personnel primarily looking for "action" do not last long in the unit: in the ironic phrase, they "burn out" and transfer.

A related issue, even for long-term workers, is asymmetry. (Indeed, this notion is important for other areas of health care and the helping professions in general.) Clearly the relationship of a doctor and a burn patient or a nurse and a burn patient is necessarily asymmetrical. The caregiver is in good health, receives pay for a professional job, can go home at night, and has social choices, weekends free, and so on. The burn patient is a prisoner of sorts (see Chapter 4), is in terrible health, has pain, has financial liabilities, has worries about the future, cannot go anywhere without permission, indeed cannot go without assistance in many cases, and certainly cannot go anywhere at all during the acute phase. Caregivers can freely question the patient's health and other matters, can inspect his or her body at will, can give orders, carry on procedures, and so on. Their role is safe, in the sense that it is structured by medical standards of care and permitted by the patient's immobilization because of dressings and/or drugs. Can we even imagine a patient taking off the doctor's pants and asking, "How did you get this scar on your knee?" Burns become an entry point into the intimate lives of patients. Skilled and humane care-givers will understand the high privilege of this intimacy and use it for healing benefit, not for personal power, voyeurism, or rescue missions.

Finally, we may discuss briefly the difficult notion of wounding to heal. In the routine discharge of their duties, burn workers inflict pain on burn patients. There is no easy way to say it: *dressing changes, hand therapy, inserting lines, and many other procedures cause pain.* Taking a patient to surgery to cut off an area of good skin to graft over a burn gives the patient a *second* wound, one that will hurt and itch considerably for weeks. One of the most dramatic versions of this paradox is illustrated by a training film about Dax Cowart, a well-known burn patient of the 1970s. Cowart was severely burned in a natural gas explosion. The film *Please Let Me Die* (1974) shows him being lowered into a Hubbard tank for debridement; "Oh God," he screams, as if being crucified. While Hubbard tanks are less used today and pain control may be better in most cases, there is still the disturbing paradox of causing harm to patients in order to help them become well. This is not a problem unique to the burn world, since many medical and dental procedures cause pain, but it appears in vivid relief in the burn unit. The wise caregiver will have his or her own understanding of this dilemma and will need to be able to impart it to patients and families. At a burn rounds one day, the consulting pediatric physician said, "We're not ready to release Rickie, not because we want to keep him, but because we don't see his family being able to give him his physical therapy. They will not be able to make him cry." By this cryptic phrase he acknowledged the necessity of harming in order to heal: Rickie's hands would not gain flexibility and strength without the stretching that would hurt him.

Metaphoric Meanings

Burns are intense, larger than life, and laden with emotions and associations. Humans try to make sense of burns with many sorts of comparisons, from the technical definitions already discussed to the images and stories we will discuss in Chapter 5. We may think of these comparisons as metaphors, interpretation of burns through comparative and evocative language (Carter 1989), bringing the inexpressible burn into meaning through words that are familiar. Metaphors typically describe difficult concepts through associational values to build a web of meanings.

In this brief section, we will look at metaphors about burns from the other direction, starting with verbal images of burns to show intensity, for example, "he burned with anger." Here burns are assumed to be intense, vivid, dangerous — known for their ferocity. With the help of the Oxford English Dictionary, we can list some traditional phrases that use burning as a metaphor for a mental state: the lover who *burns with lust*; the foolish *burning of bridges* behind one; *burning the candle at both ends*; being *branded a coward*; suffering a *bad case of burn-out*. Some issues or questions are considered "burning" (as in Alix Kate Shulman's novel *Burning Questions*, 1974). Burns can even illustrate a variety of emotions: one can burn with not only lust, but desire, envy, or rage. In each case, the root metaphor of *burn* contributes the sense of intensity, extravagance, lack of control, foolishness, or victimization. Even the *slow burn* of the actor suggests an inexorable path toward a strong emotion. Money that *burns a hole in the pocket* (or extra money: enough to burn) suggests the extravagance of the owner of the money. There are occasional bits of humorous relief, as in the Renaissance play, *The Knight of the Burning Pestle* (Beaumont 1608); here, the title indicates the erect and ardent (or burning) penis in fiery need of a pestle where it can grind soothingly. The overlapping worlds of burns and the erotic become complex, from various clichés of burning sighs to Cupid's fiery darts. To cite just one example, the lovers are "On fire" in the poem *The Wild Party* (March 1994, 93). When metaphors concretize into human behavior, we find the hot sweat of lovers during intercourse, pyromania (sexual urges satisfied by burning down buildings), and some sadomasochistic techniques, such as igniting a small amount of alcohol poured over, say, the back — even with light razor cuts inflicted first.

Over-all, the picture provided by burn metaphors shows turmoil and excess. As language helps to reveal our social consciousness, we have further evidence of the generally bad reputation of burns.

One other metaphor is an exception, however, and worth a moment's reflection: *to burn out*. Ordinarily this metaphor suggests that a person is like a fire, a light bulb, or an electrical machine that reaches the end of its power and vitality. But sociologist Ellen L. Maher has shown how the metaphor also has meanings of purgation and rebirth so that it does not seem so reductive or deterministic (1989). A burn patient suddenly entering the unit may feel the deep despair of being burned out, literally and figuratively; such a person may need insight into ways the burn experience may become a new beginning.

Burns as Defined by Our Fears

Another way to look at burns is to consider why we fear them. Some of these are commonsensical fears; after all, we say, "The burned child fears the fire." Others are irrational. Some may be either, depending on the context.

We fear pain. Probably all of us have suffered minor burns and know how sharply, how unrelentingly they can hurt. Larger burns suggest larger pains: the more surface area, the more hurt we assume. (In fact this is not necessarily true, since full-thickness burns — such as severe burns that send a patient to the burn unit — tend to destroy the sensory nerves that relay pain.) In the unit, furthermore, pain control through drugs, early surgery, and other means (such as hypnosis and imagery) has developed into an effective art. Nonetheless, all persons healing large burns will feel pain of many kinds. "Intense pain is world-destroying," writes Elaine Scarry in *The Body in Pain* (1985, 29).

We fear disfigurement. Our culture provides images of disfigured survivors, whether Captain Ahab (scarred by lightning as well as the whale's bite) or the children's story *Johnny Tremain* (Forbes 1943). Perhaps we have seen the extensive scars of a person treated before (or outside of) modern burn care; scars appear chaotic, red and white welts called "hypertrophic." With modern therapy of skin grafts and pressure (elasticized garments), such scarring occurs much less frequently, but some scars contract over joints, making normal movement impossible; these can often be reduced by surgery. On a more symbolic level, being marked, like Cain, can represent both the patient's shame and alienation and society's rejection and exile.

We fear loss of function. The badly burned person can lose physical ability or even entire parts of the body, not to mention the general debility associated with extensive bed rest. While the worst burns can do considerable damage, modern therapies can save much more function than ever possible before.

We fear destruction of our bodies (ourselves). In Tom Wolfe's book about American astronauts, *The Right Stuff* (1979), the haunting phrase "burned beyond recognition" is repeated many times, symbolic of the ultimate fear of the test pilot's wives and, of course, the pilots themselves. We all know that fire can consume — totally, utterly — that which it burns, even a human body. We deeply fear such annihilation of our bodies, the immediate homes we live in, the flesh we love dearly, the flesh that is guarded by instincts millions of years in the making. The liturgical poem "Te Deum" (sung in many musical settings) ends, "In Thee, oh Lord, have I trusted; let me never be confounded." (The Latin runs, "In te, Domine, speravi: non confundar in aeternum.") The word "confounded" carries the Latinate meaning of "melting" (as in "fondue," "foundry," and "confuse"): it means the loss of structure, as in a "melt-down." This is one of our most primal fears: to leave the world of order, support, and function, to enter a world of amorphism, anarchy, and chaos. Modern medicine can save some of the flesh formerly lost; psychiatric care can help the adjustment to new body configurations, prosthetics, wheelchairs, and other mechanical devices that may empower recovering burn patients. But even the physically fully healed patient may still face post-traumatic stress syndrome.

We fear death, especially an unpleasant, unsightly, demeaning death. With images in our minds of the burning of heretics and witches, the gas ovens of Nazi Germany, or the self-immolation of political protesters, we do not want to be *burned to death*. Such a death appears overwhelming, ghastly, inhuman: our body would be reduced to a trash fire; there is no corpse to wash, to dress, to pay respects to. A shriveling, blackening body gives us an image in compressed time of the slow oxidation that happens secretly in the grave, not in a sudden, obvious, public event.

While these five fears involve both body and mind, they have particular roots in our concepts of the flesh. The next four are related more specifically to our minds and imaginations.

We fear betrayal of ourselves by ourselves and by our tools. After all, shouldn't our cars, our heaters, our electricity always do their jobs as we need, as we expect? Homo faber (the tool maker) — that's us! A human is smart, capable, a person who fabricates at will, enjoying power and control through many tools masterfully used. Indeed, the expression "tool-using animal" has been a way of distinguishing ourselves from the other animals. To have a jolt of electricity go through our bodies is a major redefinition of what it means to be human and may make our vulnerable, animal base more clear to us.

We fear guilt and shame for "having screwed up." Who wants to appear clumsy or incompetent? Who wants to be designated by the slang phrase, "he shot himself in the foot"? Surely no one wishes to be marked by a scar, a bandage, or loss of normal movement to indicate shortcomings that appear to be moral as well as physical. Erving Goffman has written searchingly on the concept of "stigma," a mark of failure and social rejection (1963, chap. 1). Burn scars, or even grafted skin that must be protected from the sun, can stigmatize the survivor, giving him or her intense feelings of shame, self-loathing, even self-hate.

We fear the loss of our personhood, as workers, family members, functioning members of society. Especially in a society that rewards various active social roles, a person who suddenly loses such roles is unmoored, alone, and fearful about self-definition and the future. If suddenly you cannot work at the plant, bowl with your team, play with your kids, or even take out the trash — what are you worth?

We fear having lost control, annihilation, having stood next to infinite power. Just as persons who have been in automobile wrecks often hear the sounds over and over or see the sights repeatedly, so may burn patients relive the experience in slow but inevitable motion. They typically feel an overwhelming sense of helplessness and a terrifying sense of the magnitude of the force they encountered, whether flame, electricity, or chemical explosion. We are so used to controlling large machines such as cars or the power of electricity at the touch of a switch (one company advertises "the magic touch" to indicate this control) that the shock of confronting such power *directly* is a glimpse into a frightening world beyond control. When this glimpse comes, we are unprepared and overwhelmed. We fear that we will be destroyed, utterly.

When the American space shuttle Challenger blew up in January of 1986, many of us who watched the event on television at the time — or in the endless replays — feared that the crew had been incinerated in full view of the nation in a "public burning," to use Robert Coover's phrase (1977), with epic dimensions of failure and horror. The powerful engines and the highly volatile fuel should, we felt deeply, obey the commands of NASA and not burn up the highly talented and trained men and women aboard. When we saw the chaotic smoke trails, we feared "the worst." We saw pictures of the horrified parents of teacher/astronaut Christy McAuliffe at the launch and her shocked schoolchildren in their classroom watching the event on TV. They too were betrayed by this public annihilation. (The deaths, we learned later, were not from flames at all but from the trauma of the Icarus-like fall into the Atlantic Ocean.)

We fear a collection of images, from Hell to Armageddon, that symbolize the end of human time. These cultural symbols often have deep religious meaning, such as a cosmic judgment upon our souls and the end of civilization: eschaton in one form or another. Some examples are the Ragnarok of the Norse, the Götterdämmerung of the Teutons, the Day of Wrath ("Dies Irae") of the church.

Even such a provisional list of fears is formidable. Clearly we are up against a worthy opponent in embarking on this topic. Burns appear to be a point of entry into some of the most hidden, most primal areas of our minds.

What are burns? It depends whom you ask and what part of their minds they allow to speak when they answer. In a most metaphoric sense, then, burns are mirrors, because their meanings are so highly perspectival as to say as much about the speaker as about the subject being described. Michael Ondaatje's novel *The English Patient* (1993) illustrates this notion. The 1994 movie version has been very popular, in part because of the ambiguity around the patient. The title character is a burn patient in terrible shape at the close of World War II. He has no name, an appropriate state for a character who is perceived quite differently by each of the three characters circling around him — the nurse Hana, the sapper Kip, and the thief-adventurer Caravaggio. Similarly, a patient in the burn unit may be differently perceived by a nurse, a wife, and a visiting friend who saw burns in Vietnam some thirty years ago. For each person, the burns would have different associations, connotations, and meanings. Only through intense conversation could the wife and the friend realize that their underlying assumptions were radically different from the nurse's, and come to more appropriate contemporary understandings. Only through conversation could burn unit workers understand how frightening the burns were to these two visitors.

A first-time viewer of a major burn may feel ill, experience revulsion, or even pass out. A seasoned worker will understand the area, the depth, the current state of the wound, its treatment and prognosis. The highly organized, "can-do" person may see a burn as a challenge to treat, to describe, or to plumb in some fashion, perhaps in a rescue effort; if such a person sustains a severe burn, however, he or she may see a burn as something quite different, perhaps a lesson in humility. A melancholic and spurned person may imagine a burn as a potential lesson to a former lover, only to experience an actual burn as a trip to hell and yet, finally, a chance for psychotherapy and freedom.

There are two particularly negative traditions in giving meanings to burns. The first we might call "deterministic," in that meanings are received uncritically. These include images from popular culture (like the Crane story "The Monster" or the movie *Darkman*). These are dangerous because patients (or families or friends) may assume that the burn was somehow inevitable (perhaps because of the patient's personal shortcomings) and that medical personnel will be unable (or, worse, unwilling) to provide any help. In sharp contrast, the rescuer interpretation (burns are a nice challenge) can be equally unhelpful, trivializing the burns to occasions for problem-solving. By both interpretations, burns are misperceived to the detriment of the burned person and the misperceivers.

Another approach — the way of this book — is to test our associations of burns, inform them, and offer a repertory of ways to look at them, so that we can choose the ways that make most sense to us.

A final comment, then, is this: the meanings of burns are perspectival, based on the perspectives (including assumptions and associations) of the viewer. These perspectives are, however, malleable, as persons gain information and insight.

This discussion signals some of the issues we will explore in this book. Burns are serious, dramatic, and complex; they occur from many causes, some intentional, some accidental, some unfathomably strange. The healing course of burns is fraught with uncertainty, surprises, disappointments, and, often, impressive gains. Whatever else they are, burns are both frightening and mysterious. By studying what they mean, and how they go beyond logic and rational understanding, we can better grasp why we fear them, and why the burn unit is such an intense place for all who come there.

Chapter Two
Heat, Culture, and Betrayal

How do people become burned? A short answer is: by contact with something that is hotter than they are. A longer answer takes into account a wide variety of energy, both natural and human, the many ways heat is managed by cultures, and the trust we place in our heat sources. In the West, therefore, we commonly find patients burned — directly or indirectly — by petroleum products. We also see burns, whether major or minor, from barbecue coals, clothes irons, and scalding water. Each of these three sources are domestic, part of daily life in the West. We could also mention jet fuel, high-voltage electricity, open-hearth steel production, or other sources of heat in the industrial workplace. Looking outward still further, we might also think of open cooking and heating fires around the world; these are all frequent sources for burns. Even a hot sidewalk anywhere can burn the foot of a child or the cheek of an elderly person who has fallen upon it. From the natural realm, we have lightning, geysers, forest fires, volcanic lava, even the sun itself — phenomena that have held human interest all over the world. In every case, sources of heat have an ambiguous nature: they can improve our lives or destroy human tissue, even to the point of death. Sadly enough, human beings — whatever else they are — are *burnable*, and the sources of burns are many.

Humans are the ultimate tool-makers, and they especially like tools which use high energy: heat, of course, but also other forms of energy, including chemical, nuclear, and electrical forms. This involvement in energy has been — and is now — so central to our daily experience that it creates many pollutants that foul our water, air, and earth. This happens directly from smoke, particulate matter, acid rain, and carbon dioxide attacking the ozone layer, and indirectly through nuclear waste, genetic damage, and temperature elevation of the entire atmosphere. Thus we may reflect that many difficulties accompany our intense involvement with sources of heat, and burns are one of these difficulties. Humans are, for better and for worse, heat-creating, heat-seeking, heat-loving, heat-addicted animals.

The result of our love of heat sources, then, is a difficult mixture of values: we associate positive values with tools, technology, and skillful management of energy sources, but negative values with severe burns, their pain and disfigurement, and the implied betrayal of ourselves by our tools. A teenager can go to the beach expecting much pleasure, but return home with a blistering sunburn. An elderly person can enter a bathtub for a warming and relaxing bath, only to find that the water is too hot; with thin skin and arthritic joints that cannot move quickly, he or she receives a burn. In both cases, a heat source — assumed to be helpful or even friendly — inflicts harm. Besides the "insult" of the physical injury, the patient commonly suffers a feeling of betrayal or a loss of the order, justice, or benevolent nature of the world at large.

In this chapter, we will examine some of the relationships between heat and humans, and some of the harms possible through accidents. (In Chapter 3, we will turn more specifically to intentional burns, the difficult world of burns caused on purpose.)

A "Freak Accident"

A young woman in Florida was burned by electrical power lines in a strange and unusual accident. Sometimes we call such events "freak accidents" in a linguistic attempt to remove the event from normalcy, from what we expect, and from what we assume to be the basic order of the world. By labeling something as "freak" (or "monstrous") we assure ourselves that, basically, *the accident couldn't happen to us*, because it was not natural, normal, or within our understanding of risk. Any burn worker can tell us, however, that the unit is filled of victims from the "freak" accidents that happen every day. Why is this so? Because sources of heat and power surround us routinely, and when humans and heat intersect a burn results — more often than we are willing to admit.

In the case of the Florida accident,

> a young woman was using a parachute for parasailing, floating high in the air while pulled by a rope attached to a powerboat. Somehow she was blown off course by the wind and became entangled in 12,000-volt power lines. Fortunately for her, employees for the utility company were nearby. They turned off the power and removed her from her predicament with a cherry picker. A helicopter took her to a burn unit with burns over 15–20 percent of her body (*St. Petersburg Times*, 1990).

This is a strikingly modern burn, one impossible fifty years ago, since it combines the gasoline power of the motorboat with the high-voltage electricity line. Yet the image of a high flyer encountering great power is ancient. We recall the story of Phaethon, who borrowed his father's chariot of the sun and careened across the skies, out of control, until Zeus shot him down with a thunderbolt. This story, told in Ovid's *Metamorphoses* (8 C.E.), emphasizes the foolishness of youth and the punishment of the deity, not only of Phaethon but of the earth itself, since the Sahara Desert and even the dark-skinned ("scorched") people of Africa were said to be part of the result. (There are some Euro-centric values here, clearly, and some negative assumptions about deserts and various marks of Cain.) For the Florida woman, high technology participated in her fun, then her disaster, finally her rescue, and (we may assume) her healing.

Another ancient story is that of Icarus and Daedalus, a father and son who were also high flyers. We will discuss this story in Chapter 5, but for now it is enough to remember that Daedalus, the technician, made wings for escape from Crete and instructed Icarus about their use. Intoxicated by the power of flying, Icarus flew too high, so that the sun melted the wax holding the feathers and he fell to his death. This story is mythic in its wisdom, although deterministic to the point of allowing no rescue or healing for Icarus. Some modern burn patients die of their wounds, to be sure, but the vast majority survive when they receive modern burn care; in Chapter 9, we will rewrite this story as "Icarus Recovers."

In this chapter, we will explore heat sources, their relation to culture, and some of the meanings of betrayal that often accompany severe burns.

What Is Heat?

Heat appears in many forms, with many possible applications: the comfort of a hot bath, the pleasures of cooked food, the power of engines, and the beauty of fireworks, to name a few. But each of these pleasant and useful things has sent people to the burn unit. Modern, technological society is so permeated with heat and high energy sources that we are — daily, hourly — at risk for burns. Anyone riding in a car is seconds away from incineration, owing to the ever-present gas tank. Perhaps it is miraculous *that so few of us* are severely burned. Usually the risks of severe burns are relatively low, and we typically use heat in many forms without a thought to the potential danger. Culturally speaking, heat is our friend, our tool, our companion. We like fireplaces in our houses, propane grills on our patios. Power tools, electric blankets, and microwave ovens have sold extremely well in the United States. They represent ways we have domesticated heat so thoroughly that none of them seem dangerous to us. Indeed, culturally speaking, we ignore both burns themselves and even the possibility of burns. Because of such trust in the power and presumed faithfulness of heat, burns have as part of their meanings the symbolic element of betrayal, which we'll discuss in a moment.

When heat burns an individual, we consider the event unusual enough to ignore it or to marginalize it as "freak," even though a severe burn is devastating to that individual and to family and friends. Our social values regarding heat are so firmly positive, it is hard for us to think of heat as a weapon: heat is something that *works*; contrary news is disquieting, with one remarkable exception, entertainment. In particular, we enjoy the lavish use of spectacular fire in movies from *Gone with the Wind* (1939) to most James Bond movies, to *Backdraft* (1991), and many others. In such cases, fire is something spectacular that, again, happens to "other people," movie characters, and certainly not to us, the audience members.

And yet when many persons are involved in an actual burn disaster, the rest of us are simultaneously repelled and fascinated. Mass media and history accounts give thorough details of explosions, fires that consume portions of cities, and, of course, warfare. The firestorm that destroyed Dresden and the holocausts of Hiroshima and Nagasaki are among the largest examples of human-caused fires that burned, scarred, or killed outright large numbers of people (mostly non-combatants): ironically enough, it was the widespread use in Vietnam of napalm and other incendiaries coupled with efficient medical evacuation that led to many of the improvements in modern burn care. Once stabilized, burned American soldiers were sent to the Brooke Army Hospital in San Antonio, Texas, where the sheer volume of cases provided doctors with experience in which treatments worked and which did not. Once again, though, burns on a large scale appeared to be "something that happens to other people" and in other places of the world, not here.

With the Cold War on the wane, the specter of nuclear holocaust is less vivid, but for some forty-five years it was a common fear that our nations might be incinerated in an all-out exchange of nuclear weapons. Movies such as *The Day After* (1983) and *Threads* (1985) showed vivid images of heat followed by chaos, including a nuclear winter, caused by swirling ash and dust that blocked the sun's warmth. As of this writing, the threat of nuclear war is so low that people are dismantling bomb shelters put together in the 1950s. Nuclear war between the United States and Russia now seems science fiction, even though other nations and terrorist groups are serious threats.

There are also natural forces of heat that threaten us on a grand scale. Astronomers predict that the sun — arguably the source of all earthly life and much of our fuel — will eventually become a red giant and engulf the entire orbit of the earth, burning up this planet. This projected event, far distant in astronomic time, relies on the parallel evolutions of many other observed stars; it is hypothetical, of course, but an interesting and perhaps even instructive symbol of the ultimate end of the earth in flames. It also parallels mythologies that have seen the fiery *eschaton* of earthly life, such as the Germanic Götterdämmerung or the Norse Ragnarok. Even the Christian New Testament describes a lake of fire where the beast and the false prophet are to be burned up (Rev. 19.20), and Jesus' parable of the wheat and tares says that the weeds (the sinners and evil-doers) will be burned (e.g., Mt. 13.24–43). By such visions, human life and progress are not infinite: there is a fiery terminus out there for all earthly life. And yet, few people consider this end; it is too far away, too abstract, and too removed from the routines of daily life — where heat behaves as it should.

Closer to hand, we have natural forces of heat in lightning and geothermal energy (volcanoes, geysers, hot springs) that often elicit our awe and concern. A book by Norman Maclean, *Young Men and Fire* (1992) tells about the work of smokejumpers in Montana, describing in detail a group who burned to death in a forest fire started by lightning. The book sold well, not only because of the author's elegant style but because of the high drama and tragedy of the powerful flames that killed these young men.

For good or for ill, heat is a concentrated form of energy that can be transferred to humans. According to the kinetic molecular theory, this energy comes from vibrating molecules and atoms: the faster they vibrate, the more energy they have. At a certain point, such energy, when transferred to human flesh, causes harm to our cells. As we said earlier, with a great amount of heat many cells boil, explode, and steam away as vapor. But fat cells, in particular, can actually ignite: flesh and even bone can burn. (The paranormal phenomenon of "spontaneous human combustion" has even been reported, sometimes in sensational terms; a body burns away and no external forces can be identified. Ordinary fire science can almost always explain these, but various versions of the story persist, perhaps because of a human craving for mystery and wonder.) The most purposeful and efficient of human burnings is, of course, cremation; here, two to three hours of intense heat destroys all but the heaviest vertebral and pelvic bones. Everything else — organs, muscles, skin, lighter bones — goes up the chimney as hot gases. When the remaining bones are broken up, we call them "ashes," but they are really bone chips and/or powder.

What is heat? The definition depends on who is looking and with what assumptions. A chemist looks at a fire and sees rapid oxidation, or the combining of fuels such as carbon with oxygen to release energy. (Indeed the very name *oxy-gen* was proposed to indicate "the generator of brightness.") There are two major classes of oxidation: fast and slow. Fast includes fire, of course, while slow includes rust. Every one of our cells, even at rest, burns the fuel of adenosine triphosphate (ATP) molecules in combination with oxygen transported by hemoglobin in the blood. Heat is produced in minute amounts, but since we have billions of cells the net result is the stable and continuous warmth of a human being. Upon exercise, fever, or very hot climatic conditions, the body temperature rises beyond normal range. Ordinarily, the body has mechanisms to disperse extra heat, such as sweat and increased blood flow to the skin. The red spots in the cheeks of a dancer indicate the dilation of blood vessels at the surface so that the blood may release heat there, then return to cool the heated musculature. In the case of a burn, such physical strategies are immediately overwhelmed (and can be disrupted for a long time), so that heat damages tissues. In one simple definition, a burn is an injury caused by too much heat for our bodies to disperse.

According to the physicist, heat is vibration of atoms and molecules. The complete absence of heat — a theoretical state — is absolute zero (0° Kelvin). Thus all ordinary matter has some level of atomic vibration. As such motion increases, it becomes chaotic, disorganized energy, random vibrations that must be organized if work is to occur. Fire itself will not power a machine, but it can heat water to boiling, and the resultant steam can be channeled to drive a piston. In the world of burns, we can see heat as chaos: random, undirected energy that has somehow gotten loose to coincide with a person and harm the biological order.

According to a biologist, we live within a narrow range of heat, a range we are quite sensitive to, putting clothes on or off, adjusting the thermostat, or, if all fails, suffering. We are aware of differences in heat and cool comparatively, and the thermometer's reading is only one factor, along with wind, humidity, clothing, activity level, even psychological outlook. The primal event of temperature disruption for all of us was probably birth, when we left an exquisitely controlled environment for the relative chaos of the "outside world." Mother's uterus, varying less than one degree Fahrenheit, was always *just the right temperature*. It's all downhill from there, although we try, with some success, to keep ourselves in the "comfort zone," to use the architects' phrase. Besides the external manipulations of heating, air-conditioning, clothing, and the like, the body itself attempts to maintain thermoregulation through homeostatic mechanisms, such as sweat, shivering, changing blood vessel flow, or burning more food. Indeed much of our food is "burned" to keep our temperature at about 98.6° F (37° C); the reason for this apparently wasteful usage is that our temperature is usually higher than our surroundings, which relentlessly pull heat away from us. Humans give off heat at about the rate of a 100-watt light bulb: a pair of lovers in a parked car will steam up the windows; 300 persons filling a cold auditorium will warm it up.

But we also give off heat even when the surroundings are warmer than we are, simply because we are metabolic engines, running day and night. Even perspiration for cooling expends energy. Between our basic biology and our surroundings, we must find an acceptable balance, because, at the body's core, heat means life: if we are much cooler than 95° F (35° C), we begin to experience hypothermia (literally, "low heat") or exposure. If heat is not restored soon, shock and death can result. Cold temperatures can damage our skin, giving us frostbite (which is treated like a burn) or, when prolonged, can actually freeze us solid — another sense of "absolute zero," since we can't be any deader than that. In the other direction, extreme heat can cause heat exhaustion or, worse, heat stroke, when our ability to sweat and cool ourselves is entirely overwhelmed. (Victims of heat stroke do not — cannot — sweat.) The brain eventually "cooks" so that it cannot manage the nervous and endocrine controls for the rest of the body. Basically, the entire body overheats and dies. Another kind of overheating, the subject of this book, is the specific application of heat that kills tissues. The wider the application and the longer the time of it, the more danger to the life of the person. Many of the worst burns happen in enclosed spaces—garages, small workshops, below deck on small boats—where people sustain not only burns to their skin but burns to their airways and the first parts of the lung. This is sensitive tissue, readily damaged and easily infected. Inhalation injuries are treatable, but they can push a burned person over the edge, to death.

Heat, according to the laws of thermodynamics, moves from high to low, in a constant search to find equilibrium. "Heat flows downhill," is the physicist's phrase. A hot cup of coffee cools by exciting the air molecules around it, the wood molecules of the table, and the tissues of fingers, mouth, esophagus, and stomach of the person drinking the coffee. Each of the cooler substances is a "heat sink" as heat flows across the temperature differential. If the coffee is "too hot," by the biological definition of our lips, nerves will signal that our tissues are in danger of being burned, and we will pull the cup away. If we are not quick enough, our lip will be more of a heat sink than we want. A hot fondue fork, coming directly from boiling oil, can burn a lip even on the briefest contact (as one of the authors can personally attest). If we fall off a boat into the ocean, we swiftly lose energy because of the enormous volume of cooler water touching every external part of us. It's the relativity of the differences that draws the heat: you can even get the shivers on a very hot day by prolonged swimming in 90° F water; hence scuba divers in the warm waters of the Caribbean will wear wetsuits for protection against prolonged exposure. Persons burned on boats often jump overboard immediately, thereby extinguishing burning clothes and cooling burned tissues, limiting further damage to their bodies.

What is heat? Heat is energy that we define in various ways, depending on our assumptions and academic disciplines, but, for everyone, it is energy that can destroy human tissues.

Heat Sources

We turn now to more concrete aspects of burns, the heat sources that we prize for making modern life possible: engines, electricity, home appliances, and fuels of all sorts, petrochemicals in particular. Anything hot or full of energy has sent people to the burn unit; roofing tar, fires following car or plane crashes, barbecue coals, lighter fluid, boiling water, boiling sugar for candy, propane tanks, cooking oil and grease, fires in buildings, napalm, incendiary bombs, nuclear reactors, to name a few. The list is enormous, and many of reported causes of burns are bizarre. Some are ironically absurd, as in metal-toed industrial boots, certainly designed to protect the feet, but efficient enough carriers of heat to burn the toes within. Even protective high-top boots worn by metal workers have failed miserably because the workers turned them down from the knee, making a funnel for molten metal to enter and burn lower legs and feet. Sun-warmed seat-belt buckles have burned passengers instead of protecting them. Heating pads, tanning salons, and waxing for hair removal, all meant for personal pleasure or improvement, have also been sources of burns. Other sources of pleasure that have caused serious harm include fireworks, motorcycle exhaust pipes, and microwaved pie fillings.

From the natural world, there are larger sources of heat: lightning, forest fires, molten lava, even the sun itself. These suggest the cosmic or epic nature of heat and energy, fueling our fears of primal and universal powers opposing us. Television and print media enjoy showing footage of such things, which appear dramatic and large, and our instincts respond with both fascination and fear. Animals are rarely burned in the wild; they instinctively fear flame and flee from it. Indeed part of the challenge of the lion "tamer" to get lions to jump through flaming hoops is to overcome this deep-seated fear.

Another way of answering the question "What is heat?" is to ask students of culture. For a humanist, for example, heat is seen as symbolic of something else, as we saw in our metaphoric discussion in Chapter 1. Dante uses the flames of Hell for punishment in his *Inferno* (although he also uses Hell's ice). Captain Ahab's twisted psychology is mirrored by the scars on his face from being struck by lightning, and Stephen Crane's monster is assumed to be sick, crazy, or evil because of his scars from severe burns. In every case, the extremity of fire stands for extremity of emotion or moral state, and makes an individual different from normal, healthy people. Students of religion find fire widely used as a dramatic symbol (see Chapter 5). In popular culture heat can mean pressure, an intense investigation, a gun (as in "packing heat"), or a pitcher's fastball ("heater").

Heat, then, is many things, all of them powerful, and patients (and their families) may bring many associations, conscious or unconscious, about fire and burns to the hospital. As in many illnesses, it may be valuable for caregivers to ask the patient (and family), "what does this all mean to you?" Some of the values and associations will readily come forth; others may be deep and obscure, needing teasing out over time. It is worth the effort though, and patients may feel calmer and better as a result, because efforts to formulate and interpret — coupled with being listened to sympathetically — can help their psychological healing.

Cultural Aspects

Heat is a prominent tool within any human culture. Modern technological society is based on coal, gasoline, and other petrochemicals, electricity, and nuclear power. We use cars, hot water, and stoves without a second thought to their potential danger; we also take them for granted as part of our world order. When they burn us, we feel betrayal by our tools and perhaps even a collapse of our basic picture of "the rightness of things."

In third-world countries, heat is also central to life, especially for cooking. Since live flames and coals are often used (as opposed to electricity or natural gas in the West), the risk of fires is high. Saeed A. Ansari (1992) has studied third-world burns. He reports that good statistics are impossible to come by, but that the risk of fires is considerable owing to many factors: poor education, poor fire-fighting capabilities, and lack of fire safety. Much of the population is rural, with little fire protection, often not even a bucket of water near the cooking area. Living conditions are crowded, with poorly ventilated rooms that accumulate combustible and poisonous gases. Fuel is often firewood (which can smolder or shoot off fragments), kerosene, alcohol, or coal — all of which are dangerous. Women usually do the cooking, often wearing loose dress, such as saris made of flammable artificial fabrics: "saris and scarves with hanging pieces are normally the starting point of fatal injuries" (72). With low literacy rates, the populations have little concept of fire dynamics and safety. Many people smoke in bed. Ansari recommends public education about fire safety, standardization of domestic appliances, social organizations, small fire extinguishers, and first-aid kits.

Andrew Munster has studied burns in India (1994). He concentrates largely on treatment protocols and governmental infrastructure, finding that conflicts in treatment between the modern, Western methods and the traditional, ayurvedic medicine. Families often have a fatalistic attitude toward burns; they are slow to bring patients for treatment and reluctant to consent to surgery. In particular, female burn-suicide attempts (as well as burns inflicted by others on brides judged to have too small a dowry) are common and all too readily accepted.

Heat sources vary with cultures. Cooking, for example, primarily uses electricity or gas in the West but also wood, peat, kerosene, or dried dung elsewhere. Burns from cooking are universal, however, and the fuel and technology created variations on a single, sad theme. In Kashmir the portable Kangri stoves typically burned the abdomens of women, often multiple times (*International Dictionary of Medicine and Biology*, 1986). In Brazil, flame burns from alcohol used as a cooking fuel exceed scald burns — the most common kitchen burn in the United States. Even within a smaller area, say a city, burn sources will vary with the wealth of persons. Rich people have reliable heating systems in their homes. Poor people may have a space heater or even an open fire in their apartment or shack. With the first cold day of winter each year, U.S. burn units routinely expect to receive victims of fires caused by substandard heating. (Similarly, the Fourth of July will bring in burns from barbecue fires and fireworks, often with compounding factors of alcohol intoxication — regardless of social class; burn units expect to see these and plan for them.) On the other hand, it is rich persons who are typically burned from fires on pleasure boats. Sad but true: people are burned by whatever heat sources they use, but poor people, with unsafe heat sources, are often most at risk.

Blue-collar workers, for example, are more at risk than office workers. There are many burns in shops, from welding, electricity, fuels out of control, and petroleum products used in a variety of ways. A common injury results from welding a tank that still has some fuel within it, creating an explosion. In general, the more professionalized or regulated an industry, the less the risk. Well organized factories follow regulations from federal agencies (in the United States, notably, the Occupational Safety and Health Administration [OSHA]) and the directives of risk managers and other promoters of health. Often we see signs reading "This plant has 90 days without a lost-time accident." Serious burn incidents are likely to lead to changes in the conditions that caused them, for several reasons. Among these are humanitarian reasons, such as *skilled workers should not be put at risk; no one else should have to suffer*; and the like. But there are also economic and legal reasons: *we should not lose work hours or trained workers; we may get sued; our public image may suffer; our health insurance will go up*. At the same time, there are less ethically managed places, such as garment sweat shops in New York City, that may be another Triangle Shirtwaist fire just waiting to happen. An independent roofer, who hires minimally trained and often socially unstable personnel, may soon have a serious burn to deal with, and tar burns are among the worst. (Tar remains on the victim, transferring more heat. Cooled, hardened tar is difficult to remove without further damaging the patient.)

Similarly, auto mechanics in well-run garages rarely get burned, but "shade tree mechanics" with little safety training or awareness frequently come to an emergency room for treatment before referral to a burn unit. A very common burn is the "carburetor burn" (Renz and Sherman 1992). Seeking to restart an engine, a man (almost always a man) removes the air cleaner and pours gasoline directly into the hot throat of the carburetor. The gasoline ignites and flashes over in the enclosed space of the engine compartment and hood, usually burning the man's face, upper chest, and arms. (Because of wonderful reflexes, the eyes are almost always spared.) Many persons doing weekend chores, working with unfamiliar tools or materials, burn themselves. One common usage is to pour gasoline (or some other accelerant) directly on a fire "to make it burn better," a practice that brings many patients to the burn unit, especially adolescent males.

Various cultures and subcultures use heat in many ways, and each of these uses can inflict severe burns. When this happens, the victim may feel a sense of betrayal by the trusted tool. Dealing with a sense of betrayal can be a major part of a burn patient's psychological recovery.

Betrayal

In accidental burns, the patient's psychological state often relates to the cause of the burn. Typically a tool that ordinarily works well has somehow damaged the user: gasoline poured in a hot carburetor ignites, charcoal starter sprayed on a barbecue flames back to the can, faulty wiring in a house starts a fire. In each case a structure of daily life that has worked countless times before suddenly works in another way, causing a chaos of heat to harm living tissues.

Mei was preparing supper for her family, as she had done hundreds of times before. Cooking gave her great pleasure: planning the meals, buying the ingredients, and managing the dishes so that they were ready at the same time. Her family came together for the rituals of eating, sharing the day's news, and taking a break from various demands. She had decorated her kitchen in cheerful colors; she had carefully chosen and arranged all her implements.

Tonight was an ordinary evening, and various recipes were cooking on the stove. While putting ice in glasses, she dropped one cube. "I'll pick it up later," she thought, kicking it away. The cube bounced back off a cabinet, however, and slowly melted on the floor. Eventually, she slipped on the water. Falling, she grabbed for the counter. Her forearm struck a pothandle, pushing it down, and catapulting boiling soup over her face, neck, shoulder, and chest. Horrified, in pain, in shock, she collapsed on the floor, where prolonged contact with the soup on the floor caused minor burns to her legs. Her family ran to help her. No one ate an ordinary dinner that night.

Mei, of course, should have ripped away her sodden clothes and splashed cold water over herself to cool the superheated cells of her body, but she didn't. (Indeed, learning this later further depressed her during her recovery.) It has been said that all burn patients have two injuries, the injury of the physical burn and the injury of their world collapsing and attacking them—in other words, the psychological injury. In Mei's case, her world of food, her kitchen, and her family was suddenly—within a few terrible seconds—deeply damaged; the ordinarily faithful tools of her cooking betrayed her and caused grievous bodily harm. Yes, she would heal and return to her kitchen, but for several weeks before her return, she would worry about the event and its meaning, even what she had done to deserve such a terrible thing. Upon her return, she turned all pot handles to the rear without fail, a basic preventive move, an especially good idea if there are small children at home. Many small children are burned by dragging a pot handle off the front of a stove and spilling hot liquids down their arms and chests, even their faces.

Some burn patients do not remember the events of the burn, due to protective amnesia, the drugs of initial treatment, and/or the overwhelming sensations and confusion of the event. But, as they heal, they usually feel an urge to make sense of the event, to ask for information, to construct a narrative that explains the cause and includes the story of their healing. Patients sometimes ask over and over, "What happened," until they have a clear picture of the causes and events.

Sometimes they feel anger.

> How could this faithful tool betray me? How could the order, logic, even justice of the world break down and cause this great tragedy to me? I've done this a million times. Why a disaster now? Neither I nor my family deserve this!

Sometimes they feel depression:

> What's the use? If the world is going to treat me like this, why should I eat like they want here, why should I go to physical therapy?

In some cases, the burn is a result of a combination of factors, both the heat source and the limitation of the person using it.

> A man had a spinal cord injury and had lost movement and feeling in his lower body. As part of his rehabilitation, he installed a water bed in his home to avoid pressure sores. One day the water escaped from the bed as he lay on it. Asleep, he slowly lowered onto the heating element. His buttock slowly burned, but he was unaware of the wound because his lower body was insensate. Even upon waking and seeing the accident, he didn't know he had a full thickness burn. While other people helped him clean up the mess, one said, "Hey, you've got a hell of a burn on your ass," and he came to the unit. Both his bed—which was supposed to keep him well—and his body betrayed this man.

Another difficult case is this one:

> Frank and Laura were cooking supper together. Suddenly a frying pan full of grease caught on fire. "I'll get the door," Frank yelled. "You pitch the grease outside!" He ran to the door, opened it, and stepped outside. Laura grabbed the pan, ran to the door, and started to pitch it directly outward. However, she saw their brand-new boat sitting there, and reflexively avoided it, pitching the burn-ing grease to the side . . . and directly on Frank.

Sometimes it is hard to count the number of factors of betrayal and absur-dity. In this case, the grease chaotically caught on fire, a plausible plan of action failed, and finally Laura was horrified at having burned her own husband. (A wiser course, obviously, would have been to dump baking soda onto the pan where it sat, to use a home fire extinguisher, or simply cover the pan with a lid.) It took many conversations between Laura and Frank — while he healed — to relieve her of her guilt and self-blame: his physical cure was a symbolic analogue to her mental healing. Eventually, as he readied to leave the unit, they were able to laugh about the accident together. "So, the boat was more important than me, huh?" he teased. This marriage survived the burn, but others have not. Cases differ widely, but these notions of betrayal and absurdity should be discussed with patients until — if all goes well — they reach some understanding of the causes of their injuries.

The words "betrayal" and "traitor" are linked, both in their common Latin root and in their current overlapping meanings. In the example above, Laura is first betrayed by her cooking, then Frank is betrayed by the trajectory of hot grease — or even by Laura herself. In each betrayal, there is a loss of faith, first that the kitchen should work right and second that the plan to toss away the grease should solve something. We base much of our daily lives on such faiths: that the hot water should work — in a safe, controlled sort of way — the heater, the car, the kitchen, highways, factories, offices. These are all places we live and work in, places we assume will "treat us right," but also places where we could be severely burned. An extreme version of rightness and heat was the medieval trail by fire. In the Arthurian legend, when the tragic heroic Iseult must undergo such a trial, she is able to pass the test (thus hiding her adultery with Tristan) through her clever use of language. Thus she is unburned, though guilty, the opposite of colonial witches — innocent but burned nonetheless.

Absurdity is a more general term, a concept that has fascinated twentieth-century thinkers and artists. The theater of the absurd, for example, was a way of exploring the loss of meaning from the 19th century, when romanticism, positivism, Victorianism, and even some remnants of the Enlightenment (such as Newtonian physics) made it seem possible that order, logic, and progress should extend indefinitely. World War I (the "Great War"), Freud, Einstein, Marx, and even Darwin were all powerful factors challenging such an order in a great intellectual shift that gave rise to Dadaism, Surrealism, and modernism, as well as to absurdist drama. As drama theorist Martin Esslin has pointed out, absurdity doesn't simply mean chaos, it also means the loss of harmony that humans sense and fear (1969, 5–7). Sometimes middle- to upper-class patients have the most trouble with their burns: they are used to an orderly life and have a general belief system that education, hard work, cultivating relationships, and the like will assure success, particularly in building a career and gaining material goods. A severe burn may cause them to question their values, especially those they held strongly but unconsciously. They even may experience despair over "the nature of things." Some reassess their values and make changes, such as changing professions or re-evaluating personal relationships. "You have a lot of time to think in a hospital," many patients have said. Many other patients, however, even with days and weeks at their disposal, make no headway in ordering their lives.

Heat is necessary for life, but too much of it, or too little, will threaten our lives. As modern technology refines, intensifies, and proliferates the forms of heat, the risks of burns to individuals, to entire classes of people, and, in short, to all of us increases, unless countermeasures are carefully instituted.

High-rise buildings — hotels for example — can be death traps for all inhabitants as well as any rescue teams. (Firefighters frequently say that high-rise fires are the most dangerous to them personally, even in the most modern and "best" designed buildings.) On the other hand, the poorest cultures use heat for meals and warmth, uses that cause many fatal burns.

When a burn occurs, the patient will have both the tissue injury and the psychological insult — particularly of betrayal — to deal with. Skilled burn-care workers know this and have resources to meet, at least in part, the psychological harm.

Chapter Three
Burn Wounds—Damage by Accident or Intent

We have defined burns as the intersection of heat and flesh with a resultant injury, and we have looked at various sources of heat. In this chapter, we will further discuss what happens to humans as they are damaged and the various causes and intents that make burns happen. One of the difficulties in assessing meanings of burns is that burns themselves have no intentions; that is, a burn per se has no inherent reason for existence, although it may certainly result from the intentions of persons. Even if a burn does not, by itself, mean or intend any particular results, large burns always have plenty of implications (biological, for example) and the ascribed meanings from both patients and care-givers. Medical consequences, known as "sequelae," commonly include pneumonia, infections in the wound sites, and loss of body parts such as ears or fingers. Hospital staff know that an 80 percent burn will affect numerous body systems beyond the skin: large burn implies risk for burn shock. In this sense, burns may be said to have meanings, not by their own intent, but by their impact on the normal healthy processes of the body—a severe burn *means* that many body systems are harmed. (When burns are intentional—that is, caused by one person for the harm of another—symbolic meanings have yet another large dimension; we'll discuss these later in the chapter.) Because burn wounds are so dramatic, so visually arresting, so immediately evident on the body's surface, it is easy to overlook the many insults or harms burns cause throughout the body, and, indeed, much of the history of burn care has been unaware of the wider implications. Many burn patients died of burn shock and infection until those began to be understood in this century.

Our bodies function with extraordinary complexity: metabolism, heat maintenance, breathing, structural integrity, chemical balances, immune responses to pathogens, mental processes, and more—all simultaneously, all continuously day and night, and every one of these activities can be disrupted by a severe burn. The balanced coordination of these many processes has been called "homeostasis," meaning "self-maintaining balance." We might even consider that the body's central biological meaning *is* this very homeostasis: biologically speaking, the body *means* to maintain itself, its life, and its reproductive capacity at all costs. A large burn means loss of homeostasis, and, at the most extreme, loss of life.

What follows is a review of some of the body systems and processes that severe burns may disrupt.

Skin, Our Integument

Healthy skin does many wonderful things for us, most of which we take for granted; it is only when we lose its benefits that we become aware of its crucial role, much like the proverbial "worth of water when the well runs dry."

A fancy medical name for skin is "integument" ("covering") much like the husk of a seed. But our skin is remarkably flexible, allowing movement and even rapid changes in size, as in pregnancy. Our skin separates us from the world, giving us personal definition. It is also a social feature, and many of us put effort into how the skin looks in order to be attractive. When we look at our faces in the mirror, we say, *Yes, that's who I am*, and much of what we see is skin. If our faces are burned, we are deeply troubled. Skin is also a large organ, by weight the largest of the body. Depending on the height and girth of the individual, skin can equal over three square yards (just under three square meters). A large-percent burn affects much of the body, especially in children, whose surface area, compared to inner volume, is proportionately larger than in adults.

Skin is a thermoregulator, playing a major role in keeping our temperature at 98.6° F (37° C). This complex task goes on night and day, using such means as sweat and narrowing or expanding of superficial blood vessels. When skin is damaged and loses its ability to regulate heat, the whole person suffers hypothermia or heat stroke, both of which can be fatal. Burn-damaged skin cannot hold body heat efficiently. Patients whose dressings are taken down for inspection and treatment will often shiver in order to keep warm, because their skin is no longer doing the job. Burn units use heat shields, lights, and a raised room temperature to help patients maintain body temperature.

Skin is also a barrier, "the first line of defense" in the traditional phrase. Skin keeps out gross matter such as twigs, dirt, and sand, but also microscopic molds, bacteria, and viruses. It regulates water flow well and is functionally waterproof in both directions: water outside is kept there, and bodily fluids are kept inside. But skin can also be osmotic, allowing some moisture out, for example, wrinkling our fingers after a long bath. Furthermore, our sweat glands release moisture through the pores in the skin, in controlled but often large quantities. After a burn, however, a patient leaks fluid at an alarming rate and will, left untreated, die from fluid loss. This leakage—sometimes called "white blood"—is a combination of plasma from the blood, lymph, intracellular fluid, and even cellular moisture. If it goes unchecked, the result is shock or inadequate tissue perfusion: blood cannot carry sufficient oxygen to all cells; the most vulnerable cells—in the kidney, gut lining, heart, then brain—stop functioning; and the organism will die.

Furthermore, skin is an important metabolic organ, manufacturing vitamin D on exposure to the ultraviolet light of the sun. It excretes metabolic waste products (similar to the kidneys' function) through sweat. It produces antibacterial sebum, an oil that controls the colonies of bacteria normally residing on our skin. And skin, as we all know, is a tactile organ with many kinds of sensory endings that allow us to feel and to enjoy our environment, and that warn us of harm. Skin is an erotic organ, providing much pleasure in sexual activity. Skin is the first feature recognized by infants as "other" and mother, through texture, color, and smell. Lose your skin, and you lose a lot! In Chapter 8 we will look at the many modern techniques to repair and restore burn-damaged skin and to respond to all threats to other body systems reviewed below.

Burn Shock

When there is not sufficient water in the body, circulation is sluggish and inefficient; all living cells of the body are endangered. A patient arriving at the burn unit is often at risk for death by burn shock, and initial treatment revolves around fluid resuscitation. How many liters have emergency personnel already infused intravenously? How much does the person weigh? How much more fluid should be infused over the next 24 hours? These will be the crucial calculations upon which the patient's life may hang.

Immune Responses

The burn victim's immune response itself is typically depressed by the tremendous stress on the organism. Historically, victims of severe burns died from the original shock or the ensuing infections. The wounds would become septic and smelly; the patients would become feverish, and, in their weakened states, they would be hosts to massive bacterial growth, such as *Pseudomonas* or *Streptococcus,* bacilli which would spread throughout the body. Even today, different burn units have their own typical "bugs," but now the methods for identifying bugs and for treating them are sophisticated and effective. With the introduction of improved drugs, for example silver sulfadiazine (Silvadene Cream) in the early 1970s, infections became less of a problem, though always a risk. Burn staff treating patients with persistent fevers will assume that there is an infection somewhere and will try aggressively to determine its cause and location.

Nutrition

One of the more curious aspects of the physiology of burn patients is a condition called "hypermetabolism": their needs for caloric intakes skyrocket, even though they lie in bed, apparently doing nothing. A person who normally consumes 2,200 calories a day may need 6,000–7,000 per day to heal a severe burn. Various factors contribute to this puzzling condition: heat leakage because of skin damage, metabolic overdrive in burned tissues, and change in the central nervous system controlling body metabolism. Regrettably, however, the burn patient clearly cannot eat while unconscious or sedated and, even if awake, usually has little appetite. A nasogastric tube must deliver nourishment directly to the stomach 24 hours a day — and even at that the patient is likely "to fall behind" the optimal amount of calories and various components, such as protein. Thus the nutritionist is a key member of the burn team, calculating needs for each patient. Without such support, a patient can lose a pound a day, 30 pounds in a month's hospital stay. This loss is not healthy, since it comes from all body tissues, not just fat but muscle as well, even cardiac muscle, which can lead to arrhythmias. There can be further suppression of the immune system as well. Finally, calories, nitrogen, and other nutrients are needed to grow new skin and to cause grafts to adhere.

Musculoskeletal System

If the burn is very deep, muscle and even bone can be burned. The bone will not usually disappear entirely — unless the heat is intense and protracted, as in cremation — but the living cells within bone that create the structure of minerals and salts will die. Sometimes such devitalized bone can be kept in the body as an armature; sometimes it will even revitalize as living cells infiltrate. If the damage is irreparable, however, surgeons must amputate fingers or even limbs. Electric burns are especially dangerous, since the current follows the path of least resistance, destroying deep-seated muscles and even bone. Sometimes a hand will be mummified, all the moisture blasted from it — a grotesque sight. Such an extremity must be amputated. More commonly, however, the muscles and bones are not specifically injured by the burn; they are, however, at risk from disuse over the long course of treatment. Thus it is said that the physical and occupational therapists should start making their treatment plans on Day 1 of the burn: unused muscles atrophy and lose strength, unused joints lose range of motion. A patient lying on his or her back will suffer "foot drop" unless the ankle is braced; tissues contract or stretch because of the many hours in the same position, so that without proper therapy walking will be difficult or impossible in the future. Prolonged bedrest can also lead to loss of bone density, since muscles are not pulling on bones, which in turn lay down less osseous material. (Astronauts at zero gravity have the same dilemma.) Fractures associated with the burn injury (for example, a motorcycle wreck), are often hard to heal, even in a young person, because of the decreased vitality of the musculoskeletal system.

Another terrible effect is contractures of scar tissues over joints. In the past, some neck burns, for example, would result in scarring that would make it impossible for survivors to close their mouths. With modern care, these are greatly diminished through splinting and ranging (or stretching) plus surgical relief.

Respiration

We have spoken of the higher risk to patients when there is an inhalation injury, a frequent and sometimes lethal complication. The damage can come from chemical fumes (from furniture or plastics, for example). The complications for the victim can include upper airway damage (leading to swelling that can, basically, strangle the person), tissue damage to the first parts of the lung, and carbon monoxide poisoning. Damage can even reach to the most remote parts of the lung, the alveoli, those small sacs where oxygen and carbon dioxide are exchanged; when these collapse, respiratory failure develops. Lung failure caused by pneumonia or the effects of inhalation injury is currently the most common cause of death among hospitalized burn patients who survive the first few days after injury.

Other Systems

Burns can cause other kinds of havoc as well, sometimes depending on the individual. In persons with sickle cell disease, a burn can trigger a sickling crisis, so that red blood cells curl up and block circulation. Electrical burns can harm blood vessels and nerves; they can also cause arrhythmias in the heart and cataracts in the corneas, which usually come years after the burn.

Psychological Implications

This last section on sequelae will serve as a transition to our discussion of accidents and intentions in burns: patients have a lot of time in the hospital to think about the meanings of the burn event, the implications for future, and so on. These thoughts are, of course, interwoven with the patient's psychological state. We have mentioned many of these aspects already. The list by Blumenfield and Schoeps (1993) is forbiddingly long: depression, anger, numbing, anxiety, regression, denial, guilt, shame, acting out, post-traumatic stress syndrome, anxiety about self-image, paranoia, loss of self-esteem and motivation, and despair. Patients must deal continuously with pain and the prescribed analgesics, which will relieve pain but usually at the cost of dulling total awareness. Patients must deal with social isolation, loss of family and friends, loss of validation in work, and a whole set of fears, for example, loss of body parts (or function), loss of sexual attractiveness, loss of social and work roles, and loss of life itself. Some patients may develop transient organic mental syndrome, also called burn delirium or "ICU psychosis." The other major burn-related psychological disturbance occurs after discharge from the hospital; this is post-traumatic stress syndrome (PTSS), which manifests itself as sleeplessness, nightmares, irrational fears, and social maladjustments. Since this has not been well documented, its frequence and severity are unknown.

Blumenfield and Reddish have also described the psychiatric dilemma of "small burn, big problem" in burn unit patients with mild to moderate injuries but serious psychological difficulty owing to conditions existing before the injury (1987). Such patients may have sleep disturbances that continue even after discharge from the hospital. Some are phobic in response to anything related to fire or the circumstances of the injury. Some experience sexual dysfunction. Some become suicidal. The authors emphasize that these difficulties may occur with burns that are moderate or even mild. In another paper, Blumenfield and Schoeps discuss some of the pre-existing conditions that can complicate treatment of burns: alcoholism, substance abuse, diabetes, and AIDS (1993).

Beyond the specific possibilities for psychological turmoil, all patients have the daunting task of somehow making sense of the burn event, its meaning, and the healing course. For many patients there is a sense of betrayal, either of tools or of the general order of the universe, which we discussed in Chapter 2. For religious persons, the burn can raise questions about the goodness of God: how could God permit this injustice, this tragedy? This is the question German theologian Dorothee Soelle (1984) raised about the Holocaust (a word that means, at base, "burning everything"). This is the question raised in Job and retold by Archibald MacLeish in his play *J.B.* (1958). Rabbi Harold S. Kushner discusses these issues in *When Bad Things Happen to Good People* (1981) and concludes: "One reason [for bad things] is that our being human leaves us free to hurt each other, and God can't stop us without taking away the freedom that makes us human" (81). Thus we are free, in Kushner's view, to use technology, to take voluntary health risks, even to do premeditated harm to our neighbors or even entire populations, because God (or fate, or happenstance, depending on your point of view) allows this. Kushner believes, however, that God sides with the victims: "I have to believe that the Holocaust was at least as much of an offense to God's moral order as it is to mine." For some burn patients and their families, God's presence becomes clearer during the long time of healing from a severe burn. For others, a burn may be further proof of the inhospitable or even malevolent nature of the universe.

We have reviewed some of the body systems threatened by severe burns. Most or even all systems are at risk regardless of the original causes of the burn accident: a burn patient will be hypermetabolic no matter what the burning agent or the reason for the accident. The last category, psychological sequelae, however, may vary widely with the patient's condition at the time of the burn and whether the burn was accidental or intentional.

Accidental Burns

At burn rounds one day a resident remarked, "Behind every burn there's a stupid story." The other residents chuckled and shook their heads at the sad truth of this remark. Even an attending physician quipped, "Ain't that the damn truth!"

The more we look into the world of burns the more we are struck with the absurdity of burn events. In theory, every single burn was preventable, perhaps even *easily* preventable: from a rational point of view, not a single patient *should* be in a burn unit. But burns are not rational, nor do they fit into a general social vision of order, control, logic, and other values we prize in the technological West. For this discussion we will distinguish accidental burns from intentional ones, although even in the accidental burns there may have been intentions, usually in other directions than burns. And even in clearly intentional burns, there are results that the "burner" never could have intended. The following case illustrates some of these points.

> Frank didn't like the grass that grew right next to his workshop. He ran his lawn mower as close to the wall as possible, but there was always a narrow strip of grass left. He didn't have a weed trimmer, and he was unwilling to spend time on his hands and knees for slow weeding by hand. Knowing that gasoline kills plants, he began to pour a thin stream along the wall of the building, walking backwards and turning corners with care. He was about half finished when the air-conditioning unit on one side cycled on. A spark from the unit ignited gasoline fumes that rose from the ground, and flames coursed first downward to the ground then outward in two directions along the building. One branch of flame went harmlessly to the point where Frank began. The other branch rounded the corner and shot quickly toward him. The fire ran up the stream of gasoline he was pouring and exploded the can. Flaming gas sprayed over him and ignited his clothes. He rolled on the ground to extinguish the flames. He was brought to the nearby burn unit with a major burn, both by area and by depth.

In this story — told with some awe by emergency personnel — Frank attempted to use gasoline for a specific goal of caring for his workshop and yard; his intentions were to improve his property. His values were neatness, order, and efficiency. Gasoline is, of course, the wrong tool, although it might have worked, however crudely, since gasoline pulls moisture from vegetable matter, killing it. In this case, one high-energy source, gasoline, was ignited from a chance intervention with another high energy source, electricity. The timing was critical: if the air conditioner had started up before Frank passed by, there would have been no harm. If it had started up after the initial heavy fumes dispersed, there would have been no harm. And so it is with a million stories: a few seconds one way or the other, a few inches so that the pot handle on the stove was not struck by a hand, a few feet so that the hot grease did not hit the husband. And yet we tell stories of burns as cautionary tales, with an implied judgment; the paramedics speaking of Frank's injury, for example, implied that such a thing would never happen to them because they would never use gasoline that way, that such a thing was perhaps deserved by Frank—clearly a scapegoat—because he was so stupid. Not only do we seek to warn ourselves against such stupidity, we also separate ourselves as clearly smarter and therefore not at risk for accidental burns.

But, of course, people burned by accident never intended to be stupid or to be burned. Most would have no idea what is involved in a major burn or the intensity or length of the healing; even if they had such knowledge, an accident could occur anyway. A lot of smart people come to the unit as the result of accidents. Sometimes a patient's smart response can, however, limit the burn.

> Lou Anne was cooking in her apartment, stirring a pot on the back burner, when her sleeve caught fire from a front burner. She looked in horror at the flames, but immediately thought: Stop, drop, and roll—a motto she had learned at school years before. She tossed her spoon aside, dropped to the ground, and rolled over to suffocate the flames. Her burn was smaller in size and depth than it would have been otherwise.

One way of discussing accidents is in terms of risk. By using gasoline inappropriately, Frank greatly increased his risk for an accident. Anyone spraying lighter fluid in a barbecue raises the risk of burning tremendously. But specific numbers cannot be worked out, and even approximations have no predictive value. There are, for example, numbers for car accidents per passenger miles, but some people have many wrecks while others have none. Some people clean paint brushes with gasoline routinely with never an accident, while others are burned simply because they were "in the wrong place at the wrong time," like a woman who walked into her garage at the exact moment a water heater pilot light ignited fumes from a gas can, flashing over the entire garage.

We think of accidents as random, contingent, having no real cause. This formulation helps relieve us of responsibility: we say it was "just an accident," or even "a freak accident." And yet, every burn has a cause, and every cause could have been avoided. Some children walk through coals left on the ground from a charcoal fire, sending them to the unit for burns on their feet; obviously those coals could have been more safely discarded, for example by having the melted ice from the cooler poured over them. We will return to social aspects of prevention in Chapter 10.

Survivors of burns usually spend a lot of time assessing the causes of the burns and their own personal roles in the events. If they assess the burn as an accident, they wonder how it could have been avoided, or even whether the world itself is cruel and unjust. Some patients may see the burn as an act of fate or even a judgment on them. Some may decide that the burn was an accident, but a good accident. Now and then a young man living a slap-happy, high risk life will come to the unit and use the time for self-assessment; he may decide to go back to school or to marry a long-term girlfriend, particularly as she faithfully visits the unit. He may heal broken family relationships or decide "to make something of myself."

Some patients injure themselves through high risk behaviors, such as driving cars or motorcycles while intoxicated or drug-impaired, or through careless use of firecrackers, toy cannons, and petroleum products. One youngster was pounding gunpowder into a small cannon when an explosion gave him a 40 percent burn. For some patients such a burn is a lesson, and many of them are very careful with anything resembling the cause of their burn for the rest of their lives; some are even extremely afraid of cars, planes, heaters — whatever the cause — and may need counseling to mitigate this phobia. Others, however, seem to be high-riskers for ever. One patient won a huge settlement from a burn injury and went out and bought a fast motorcycle with the money. While some observers like to feel that burn patients are routinely "improved" by their injuries, our experiences suggest that more patients have a tragic, cynical, or passive view of life.

There are many kinds of accidents and many kinds of responses of patients to their misfortunes.

Intentional Burns

Some of the saddest and most depressing stories of the burn unit involve intentional burns. In these, someone desired to cause harm to someone by a weapon of flame, chemical, or other means. It is hard to imagine the amount of emotion — be it hate, wish for vengeance, or desperation — that would motivate such actions, but burn units see many intentional burns. In this section, we will discuss burns to other persons first, then burns to oneself.

Anita was tired of her husband running around and coming home drunk. She would wait up for him and berate him, but he was usually too intoxicated to pay attention. Sometimes he would flop down on the living room sofa and gesture for her to leave him alone. This night she had been cooking grits in a large pot. She poured the boiling mess onto his face and neck, then over his crotch.

This kind of burn is fairly common, although the agent varies. When women burn men, food is often the weapon: sometimes stew, sometimes grits, sometimes just boiling water. (Food that is sticky is especially effective in holding heat to the tissues, and hard for burn personnel to clean off.) When a man burns a woman, the agent may be battery acid or lye. In either case, the most common reason is revenge for sexual infidelity; indeed, such punishing burns are often well known within some subcultures as the appropriate response. The intentions include punishment, revenge, and expression of frustration and hatred at a new level of intensity. The harm to the burn victim, we may suppose, is intended to be proportionate to the psychological harm to the attacker, somehow equal to the betrayal, shame, and lack of attention. If the head is attacked, mutilation of attractive good looks may be an intention. If the genitals are attacked, the intentions may include mutilation or even destruction of the organs of betrayal. In Latin and South America, alcohol is a common fuel for small cooking stoves. Sometimes it is also used to splash on an enemy or lover in order to ignite him or her. In one case, a woman was doused and ignited by her jealous boyfriend, giving her a 60 percent burn. After her treatment she became not only a burn-care worker but also a social activist working to change the laws that protected her assailant from prosecution.

Child Abuse

Another common burn, human against human, includes the burning of children by adults. These are some of the most tragic burns, emotionally hard for medical personnel to treat, especially if they are parents.

Sally brought her two-year-old boy to the emergency room. She was agitated and distraught. "It's just a fever, and he won't eat," she kept repeating. And: "You don't really need to look at him." The staff were immediately suspicious, having heard such things before. They disrobed the child, and found a large burn on the child's buttocks and genitals. They noted in the chart "wounds consistent with being dipped into hot water." Further examination revealed cigarette burns on the soles of his feet. The child was treated and turned over to the child protection team of the hospital. The live-in boyfriend was eventually charged with the abuse.

Cases of this type are frequent (some 10 percent of children admitted to burn units have been abused by burning). Often it is a male, poorly bonded to the children, who has caused the harm. He may be a father, a boyfriend, a relative, even a babysitter, and the burn is the result of a combination of emotional tensions and lack of parenting skills and attitudes. Sometimes the burn is nominally intended to punish the child for crying, for wetting the bed, for soiling clothes, or, more generally, for disrupting the relationship of the man and the mother. Sometimes other factors have built up frustration and diminished control, such as lack of work, drinking, even the chronic poor health of a child who cries a lot. Child-abuse burns are reported most often among lower socioeconomic classes where child-care is often limited or absent, but such burns occur in every social stratum. Children of well-to-do families are also intentionally burned; sometimes they are privately treated, never reaching the burn unit or, therefore, national statistics.

As in the burn of the sleeping man described above, there is also a "tradition" of burning young children to somehow punish and improve them. A unit will see this crime again and again; it is a learned behavior. One factor is generational: an abused child sometimes grows up to abuse his or her own children. Another is subcultural: often the received knowledge is that burning is an appropriate punishment for, among other things, lapses in toilet training. Dipping the child in hot water is a grotesque parody of a cleansing bath, an event that ordinarily should bond parent and child more closely. Emergency room workers figure that burns from the bath are accidental and caused by the child if the foot is burned and scattered burn areas appear in splash patterns. By contrast, burns caused by an adult are buttock and genital burns with a clear, straight demarcation between burned and healthy flesh, caused by dipping the child into the hot water. Another common indicator of abuse is the "glove" or "stocking" burn to arm or leg, a circumferential burn with, again, an even border between injured and well skin, indicating that an adult plunged the limb into hot water, typically as a punishment. As for cigarette burns, only the adult could be guilty in most cases. Tragically, these wounds are seen again and again.

Other Attacks

Staples of lurid detective fiction have included acid thrown in the face, cigars ground out in the face, and other torturous burns. While such attacks happen, they are uncommon, more alive as social images than as common occurrences. Sometimes persons sleeping in parks are set on fire. As mentioned above mothers-in-law in India sometimes push their son's new bride into a cooking fire because her dowry was insufficient. David Rothenberg was burned when his father set his room on fire (Rothenberg and White 1985). Other examples of attacks on property include, of course, arson. Fire, however, is a difficult weapon for a single person to control. The most efficient and terrifying uses of fire as a weapon have been large-scale military uses.

Intentional Burns on a Larger Scale

Some events have been reported in mixtures of history and folklore. The emperor Nero, for example, has been portrayed as the cruel and hedonistic emperor who fiddled while Rome burned; he is said to have set on fire the sections of town he wanted to rebuild, with no regard for the citizens living there. Whether true or not, this story suggests the arbitrariness of large fires, roaring uncontrolled, killing at random. Similarly, in warfare fire has often gone out of control, killing civilians or even soldiers on the same side. One of the most memorable images of the Vietnam war is Nick Ut's photograph of a girl running from napalm (see Figure 12, Chapter 6). When the burn was personalized, when the girl was shown naked, running, and screaming, the war took on new horror for thousands of Americans.

The firestorm at Dresden similarly became a symbol for the ferocity of World War II, but only in later years. The Allies bombed the city heavily, creating a firestorm that killed 135,000 people, even though the town was not a military target. Kurt Vonnegut's novel *Slaughterhouse Five* (1969) and Vincent Ward's film *Map of the Human Heart* (1993) both portray this event and explore the horror of it. Wartime devastation by fire of persons, their towns, and their artistic heritage is something we — and our artists in particular — are still assessing.

The murder and burning of Jews and others by the Nazis has been much described. According to Robert J. Lifton (1986) the psychology of the Nazi physicians allowed them to justify mass murders as a purgation of unhealthy elements in the German race, a kind of mass cautery or, in his phrase, "killing as a therapeutic imperative" (15). The killings — by gunfire, injection, or gassing — left thousands of cadavers. Some were bulldozed into mass graves, but many were burned in crematoria, a "technical solution" to a "technical problem" (176–78). The images of the fires, smoke, and stinking residue remain painful for many; Thomas Keneally's *Schindler's List* (1982) and Steven Spielberg's Oscar-winning film based on it (1993) are recent expositions of this dreadful era.

Cremation has a long tradition, although some moderns have been aversive to it — in part because of marketing by the funeral industry, which finds better profits in standard burial. Although using huge amounts of gas, cremation is one of the least expensive ways of disposing of a body. Gas ovens running at some 2,000° F can burn up a body in two to three hours, leaving only fragments of the heaviest bones, the lower vertebrae and the pelvis. Everything else — fat, muscle, bone — goes up the chimney as smoke. Fat, of course, burns particularly well and helps the initial burning of the body.

Probably the most famous (or notorious) tradition of burning persons not dead nor even sick is the practice of suttee, now illegal in India. Upon the death of a husband, the wife was burned along with his dead body. (To say casually that she was "burned alive" cannot be technically accurate, since she would have died of suffocation first in the oxygen-starved air, but clearly she was put to death by fire.)

Suicide by Fire

In the United States, suicide attempts by burning are not as common as drug overdoses, but a burn unit will likely see several a year. They do not, however, turn out as a simple "cry for help" and a short hospital stay, since damage is usually considerable and most are fatal, at the scene, in transit, or later in the hospital. Once again we have a culturally learned behavior. Perhaps the dramatic aspects of the action make it glamorous, newsworthy, and — literally — flamboyant. Reasons can vary from problems in love (very common) to social protest, as for some Buddhist monks and others who immolated themselves during the Vietnam conflict.

A typical case of a disappointment in love might run like this:

Muriel had rejected Orrin once again—for the last time, she said. There were bitter words. "You'll be sorry," was the last thing Orrin said to her. He drove home and drank heavily. Then he siphoned gas from his car's gas tank into a plastic bottle and drove back to her house. Pausing nearby, he poured the gasoline around his car's interior, then drove over the curb and crashed into her front door. He lit his cigarette lighter and watched the flames go up. Firefighters put out the fire and paramedics took him directly to a nearby burn unit, where he lingered for two days before dying of his extensive wounds, including inhalation injuries.

Often there is an impulse for the grand gesture, the fireball which will somehow symbolize the depth of hurt in the rejection and, *finally, really get the other person's attention*. The person who did the rejecting should somehow see the true consequences of the rejection and feel sorry for the person burning up in his or her sight. One woman was so emotionally distraught that she had the specific aim of burning off her breasts to make clear to the man how much he had mistreated her. Like jumping from famous buildings or bridges, self-immolation because of unhappy love affairs is a culturally known event, a ready-made symbol that awaits gasoline and match.

Political and Religious Immolations

Self-immolation for political protest is also well known as an event, but it is usually so completely done that there are few survivors. While fellow protesters can explain the politics involved, the charred cadaver cannot share any psychodynamics with burn workers. Nonetheless, such an event is usually well covered by mass media since it is public, dramatic, and spectacular. As observers, we feel compelled to look; our eyes are forced to the spectacle of a fellow human being going up in flames; the horror is hypnotic: it is impossible to ignore or forget it. Many thoughts run through our minds as we grope for rational explanations. Was this person crazy? How did he or she manage to have the mental strength to go through with it, to go beyond the all-powerful human instincts for survival? Was there much pain? How soon did death come in the super-heated air that enveloped the body? (Fire science tells us that death comes very quickly from asphyxiation by hot gases rising up the body to mouth and nose; see Appendix 2.) What separates those of us who are still alive from persons who have burned themselves?

Probably the most widely described and photographed immolations in recent decades were the series of Buddhist monks who burned themselves in protest of the war in Vietnam. These events "played well" in the press, since editors found the pictures dramatic but, at the same time, personal (see Figure 13, Chapter 6).

Less dramatic burns among Buddhists in the Mahayana tradition of Japan have been reported as well, ritual burns on the arm, roughly 1 percent TBSA (Budny et al. 1991, 335–37). Caused by prolonged contact with incense, the burns seem to be symbols of spiritual advancement toward Nirvana and are conceptually based on *The Threefold Lotus Sutra*, which describes a monk who burned himself as an offering of his own body. Among some American college fraternities, burns have figured in initiations as brands that serve as a rite of passage and a mark of inclusion in the subgroup. The resultant scar tissue from such burns may, however, cause the wearers trouble in later life.

In the fall of 1994 several dozen religious cultists died in Switzerland and Canada, primarily from bullets and suffocating plastic bags, although the fire that followed may have finished the lives of some of them. Part of the apocalyptic imagery they appeared to share with similar groups (David Koresh's Branch Davidians of Waco, Texas, for example) was that a final fire would consume their houses, belongings, and bodies, because the end of the world was indeed at hand. The image of the Swiss and Canadians became confused, however, as evidence of illegal activities emerged. To outsiders, the meanings of the fire rapidly became less religious and more criminal.

Arson in many forms has been a hope for criminals seeking to cover their tracks, to cash in on insurance, or to create a large public event. For some there is a psychosexual thrill; indeed, police often search crowds drawn by the fire because pyromaniac arsonists who stay to see the large, public fire can often be identified — frequently they "wet their pants" from the sexual excitement. An increase in fires of a suspicious nature within communities served by volunteer firemen often suggests that there is an arsonist-fighter at work.

Conclusion

At the corporeal level, burns are dangerous for many reason. Burns destroy or damage our skin, the miraculous garment that encloses and protects us. They also cause sequelae that can kill us, such as burn shock and infections. In the long, difficult process of treatment and recovery virtually every body system is affected, including the psychological state of the patient, which may be complex because of underlying conditions and/or the causes of the burn, whether by accident or by intention. After the acute phase of treatment, burn patients have much time to ponder the meanings of the burn and event, especially in larger contexts of causation, justice, even transcendental implications. In short, humans regard burns as ferocious for many good reasons, including the severe damage they may do to body and mind. From a medical standpoint, burns are an opponent of heroic stature, and these wounds occur, furthermore, from myriad causes, both accidental and intended. Agents of burns vary with the uses of energy within cultures, and modern, high-tech societies have a wide range, from electricity to petrochemicals to radiation; traditional cultures, however, are also rife with burns, even from simple wood fires for cooking and heating. Especially for intentional burns, burns vary with traditions of punishment, from suttee to burning of witches, from burns inflicted on lovers to self-immolation. Intentional burns, whether small scale for a ritual brand or large scale as in war, are especially disturbing to the burn survivors, their family and friends, caregivers, and the public at large.

Chapter Four

Prison or Nursery? Patients' Limitations in the Burn Unit

A person burned enters a series of restrictions that bear a strong resemblance to going to jail. Some of these limitations are, of course, physical, while others are psychological, social, and even spiritual. We will discuss here restrictions that are intrinsic to modern burn care. (We leave to the side arbitrary restrictions of bureaucrats, unit directors, or anyone else; these of course should be halted.) But even the restrictions of standard care are oppressive to patients and should be mitigated — if only through humor — as much as possible. Family, friends, and of course the actual patient can benefit from frank attention to the various imprisonments of a severe burn and ways to diminish them.

Healthy, mobile people take for granted the ability to move: to put on shoes, to walk out the door, to drive a car. Put such people in a cast or on crutches, and their balance changes, their ranges of motion diminish, and, consequently, they lose their sense of freedom to move, to travel, or in general to put their wishes into action. Such movement and attitudes make up much of our sense of what it is to be human; take them away, and self-confidence and self-esteem can plummet. Any sense of agency now or in the future is threatened. Depression can become as formidable an enemy as the burn injury itself. Such mental attitudes become part of the imprisonments of a burn patient, right along with the bandages, the intensive care, the limitations of visitors. The purpose of this chapter is to describe these imprisonments and to discuss how they may be recognized and, if possible, eliminated or at least limited. A counterpointing metaphor for this chapter is that of the nursery, a concept already introduced: symbolically a burn patient undergoes, for better and for worse, a second infancy.

From the instant of a severe burn, the patient's life is radically changed, circumscribed by a series of enclosures. The body itself is limited by blisters, dead skin, and scar tissue; the patient enters the web of emergency care,

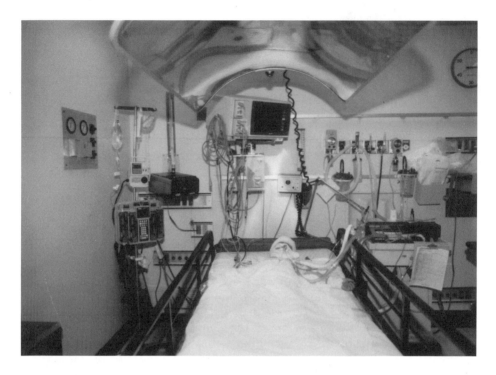

Figure 4. "Medical prison." A burn patient in an intensive care bed in the burn unit of Westchester County (New York) Medical Center. The head shield over the bed warms the patient during dressing changes; the monitor hanging from the wall over the bed displays readings of blood pressure, cardiac function, and intravascular pressures from catheters placed in the heart; the ventilator to the right breathes for the patient.

bandages, and hospital walls; social contacts are profoundly disrupted. As the patient gains consciousness and awareness, the mind keenly feels these limitations and their cumulative effect. Besides all the mechanical enclosures, the mental ones can be overwhelming: delirium, denial, despair. The metaphor of imprisonment is dramatic, extreme. Is it too exaggerated a concept to apply to severe burns? There are, of course, differences between the two worlds: guards and wardens rigorously keep convicts for a specific sentence, carefully denying possible escapes. Health-care workers seek the earliest practical release of their patients—at least in theory. (Some burn units even release patients prematurely, often because of funding and other bureaucratic pressures.) Prisons are meant for punishment (and sometimes rehabilitation), while hospitals seek to relieve pain and suffering and, aggressively, to begin careful rehabilitation of their patients. Prisoners typically have the same experience week after week, while patients (unless they die) generally find a healing course and, week by week, experience variety in their condition, treatment, and prospects. Follow-up care from both prison and hospitals, however, is usually poor.

What, then, is the value of using the metaphor of imprisonment? It can direct our attention to the loss of freedom of the burn patient and the feelings of degradation and punishment as he or she lies isolated in a burn unit. Especially in Western, industrial societies, many of our highest values cluster around concepts of freedom, action, movement, and doing. To lose these is to lose a lot. We argue that by better understanding the metaphor of imprisonment, burn-care workers may gain increased sensitivity to the experience of burn patients (see Figure 4).

While the main thrust of the chapter will be the prison metaphor, the countervailing image of the nursery provides equally suggestive insights and is, furthermore, a source of hope. Burn patients are like infants in their helplessness; nurses, like parents, must feed, change, clean, and comfort these patients, who, especially in their acute phase, cannot talk or indicate wishes — let alone take care of themselves. (The parts of the word "infant" literally mean "non-speaking.") Because of the helplessness of burn patients, the unit has some similarities to the nursery, and some patients clearly regress to an infantile state. Others, with good reason, rebel against these limitations. Again, there are differences: the adult burn patient has a mind already formed, a mind that interprets the burn experience against his or her life experience, a mind that wants to return to normal life. There also may be some negative values to identify and soften, such as possible condescension by staff or visitors to a patient's passivity and apparent or actual loss of all responsibility.

Various Imprisonments

The first and continuing imprisonment is the new condition of the physical body which has been harmed. As the patient enters the medical world the body floats between the two worlds of the patient and the hospital, owned by neither, sought for by both. A patient who suffers a major burn is immediately a prisoner of a very large wound over his or her body. If the burn is full thickness, the tissues remaining are stiff and dry, and a thick substance called eschar forms over the wound. This tough dry covering is dangerous because bacteria can grow in and beneath it, endangering the patient. Some wounds cause so much swelling that a limb becomes tight to the point of shutting down blood vessels; in such cases surgeons will make a long cut (an "escharotomy") down the limb to relieve the compression (see Figure 5).

Even with lesser burns, there are similar imprisonments and treatments to free the patient. In partial thickness burns, superficial layers of skin blister up. When they break, they leave scraps of dead skin that look like curled up leaves partially detached from the patient's remaining skin. Some-

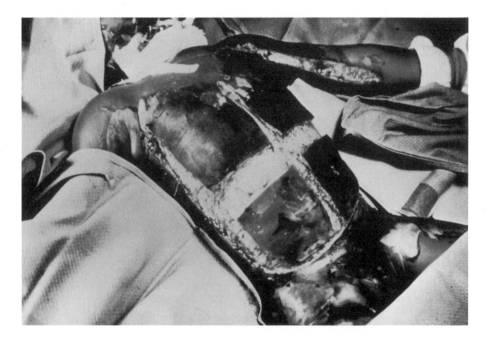

Figure 5. Escharotomy. Deep burns immediately become firm and stiff, like leather. When they go completely around the chest or an extremity, the swelling of the underlying tissues causes pressure that can restrict breathing or circulation. Intentional cuts into the burned skin, called escharotomies, relieve that pressure and prevent catastrophic complications.

times such dead skin is held by its edges, extending out like little brown flags. Such scraps are dangerous, since they harbor bacteria that can make wounds septic and eventually kill the patient: hence the treatment known as "debriding." (The French origin of this word means "bridle," as for a horse; in debriding a wound, we remove the bridling or limiting flesh.)

Debridement

From the patient's point of view, debridement is a nasty experience. There are various methods, but commonly it runs as follows. First of all, the patient will know that debridement is scheduled and will dread the day, the hour. Nurses give the patient a heavier than usual dose of pain medication, which will be successful only in part. The patient is transferred from bed to a stretcher — often a painful process in itself — and wheeled to a debridement room. (Sometimes this room is purposefully distant, so that other patients do not hear yells and screams.) The patient is transferred to a slanted stainless steel table, flowing with warm water. Often there is a heat lamp overhead, but temperatures are impossible to control for total comfort. Nurses, masked and gowned, cut off the bandages, stripping the patient naked in order to assess and treat all wounds. They may use scissors, forceps, sponges, or other tools to clean, trim, scrub, or otherwise separate dead flesh from living flesh. Surviving nerve endings wildly signal pain. The patient may call (or yell or scream) for more medication. The nurse will check the chart to see how much has already been delivered before injecting more into the IV. (One of the grislier accounts of debridement in a Hubbard tank is in the film *Please Let Me Die* about patient Dax Cowart — discussed below. In this graphic film, debridement appears as torturous as a crucifixion.) Not only are Hubbard tanks now less used, but some of the more difficult debridement are now carried out under total anesthesia; the nurse can scrub briskly and thoroughly with no immediate pain to the patient. Later, however, the skin will signal its pain.

Scar Tissue

Much later in the course of treatment, the healing skin may create a large amount of scar tissue. Left untreated, this may appear as hypertrophic scars, the kind of deformity that was typical of burns over the history of humankind until modern treatment, the kind of deformity that made burn survivors appear as freaks or monsters (see Figure 6a). In addition to the unpleasant visual aspect, the loss of movement for patients can be profound. If the front of the neck and upper chest are burned, for example, the resultant scar tissue can cause such contractures that make closing a mouth impossible. Scars on a woman's shoulder make it hard or impossible for her to fasten a bra behind her back even after she is considered "healed."

Modern pressure therapy has done much to avoid such scars, but the elastic garments themselves have an imprisoning aspect (see Figure 7). Such garments are prescribed for up to a year, to be worn 23 hours a day (one hour out for bathing). At the burn clinic one day, an athletic man asked, "Hey doc, how long do I have to wear these damn things? I'm back on the job — outside, you know? — and I soak these through in the first hour."

"I know," the physician replied, "they don't breathe worth a damn, but if we don't keep pressure on your skin for another six months, your skin won't look good for the rest of your life."

Persons burned on the face look especially strange with pressure garments; even if the rubberized fabric is skin-tinted, it still looks like a bandit's mask. If there is a mouth appliance (to prevent a contracture called "microstomia" or "small mouth"), the visual appearance is even more bizarre. Some patients wear sunglasses or a hat to minimize these odd looks, but they still receive stares with their own isolating or imprisoning effect. For a long

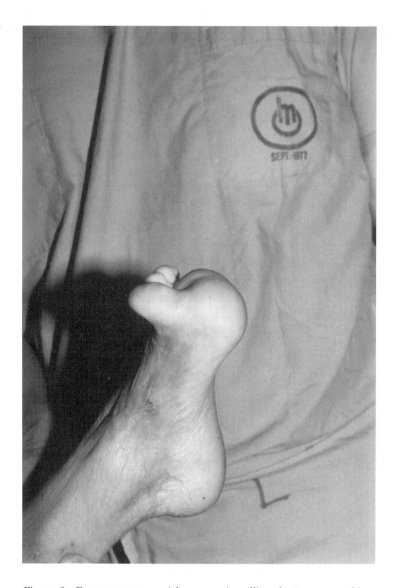

Figure 6a. Foot contracture. A burn scar is pulling the toes up, making it impossible to walk properly or wear shoes. Such contractures result from prolonged healing and were common before early skin grafting, splinting, and physical therapy became standard practice. Failure to wear pressure dressings after initial healing may also result in contractures as the burn scar thickens. Fewer than 10 percent of burns treated in a burn center will develop contractures. Photo by Jane Arbuckle Petro.

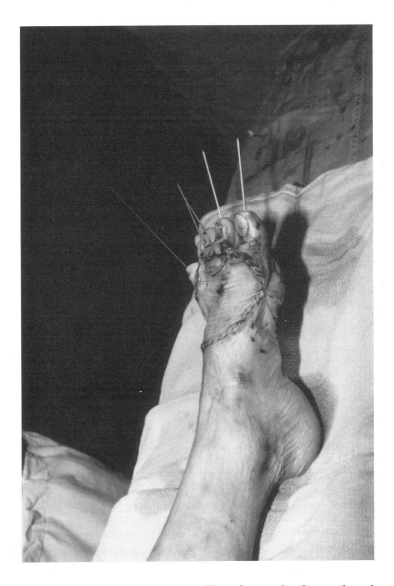

Figure 6b. Contracture treatment. Here the scar has been released and the resulting opening covered with a skin graft. The pins hold the toes in their proper position. After prolonged contracture the joints may also need reconstruction. Photo by Jane Arbuckle Petro.

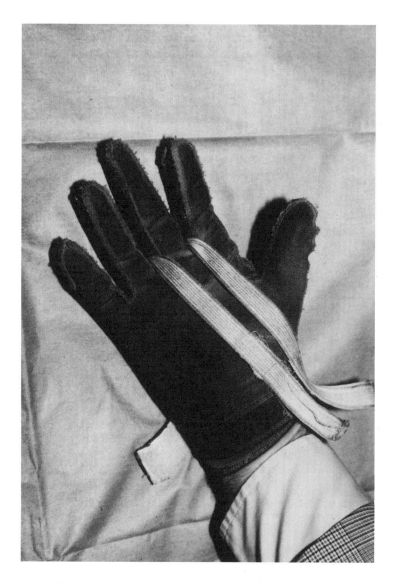

Figure 7. Compression glove. This glove, manufactured by Jobst, Inc., keeps pressure on collagen fibers so they lie flat while they heal. Otherwise thick scarring can cause contractures. The patient must wear the glove 23 hours a day, perhaps for six months. Photo by Jane Arbuckle Petro.

time, dark-pigmented patients suffered the strangeness of wearing pink-colored garments, presumably because manufacturers did not believe the market for darker garments was large enough to justify the expense.

Clear plastic or acrylic masks are sometimes used for pressure to the face; these have the advantage of allowing natural features to show through, although the total effect is unusual and upsetting to some people. For the burn patient, the masks are hot and, symbolically, oppressive or, once again, imprisoning.

Other Limiting Devices

So far we have been considering only damage at the surface — "superficial" in the medical sense, although, of course, profound in any personal sense. The picture is even grimmer if the damage goes deeper into the body, for example, broken bones, charred muscle, or electrical damage to deep nerves. Since ordinary plaster or fiberglass casts cannot be used over burned skin, surgeons may stabilize a broken arm with eternal fixation devices, metal pins that stick out from the arm and are connected to what looks like an Erector-set configuration. A patient looking down at an arm or a leg with such devices sees an alien armor, spidery prison bars that appear to grow out of or stab into the flesh. Certainly such devices may also suggest future healing — and health-care workers usually explain and repeat such values — but the limitation of freedom for that limb and that patient is, like many other symbols of the burn world, abundantly clear.

Perhaps the ultimate in loss of physical freedom is the Stryker frame, a large contraption that suspends (and can rotate) the totally immobile patient. Patients who are conscious typically hate this device and can even lose sanity while in it. (The film *Darkman* portrays the burned protagonist on a variation of this upright bed in a kind of crucifixion.) It is now rarely used, largely replaced by air-flotation beds.

During acute treatment, the patient may have a ventilator tube down his or her throat, a nasogastric tube for feeding, a urinary catheter, and one or more IV lines, as well as heavy bandages, splints, and other mechanical hindrances. The drug regimen will include analgesia for pain, of course, but often as well a muscle relaxant that will cause paralysis so that the patient will not "fight his vent" in the hospital phrase. As consciousness increases, so will the patient's sense of being imprisoned and (usually) the desire for freedom. Sometimes rebelliousness is a factor: sometimes patients pull their own tubes out. In Brian C. Clark's play *Whose Life Is It Anyway?* the central character is a trauma patient; somewhat obstreperous, he refers (in the 1981 movie version) to consciousness-limiting drugs as a "pharmaceutical nightstick." The corresponding term in physician-nurse slang is "chemical chains" or "chemical restraints."

Social Aspects

Much has been written about the enclosing nature of medical treatment, entering the "patient's role," and the like. We will focus here on some of the specifics of trauma care and, of course, burn care. Typically burn patients arrive at the burn unit by two routes. The first—and less common—is transportation by family, friends, or a good samaritan. The injured person may be curled up in the back seat of a car, holding his or her head, or have the arms crossed over the chest. Whatever the position, the patient has already lost the ability to sit up normally. Occasionally, severely burned persons will drive themselves to the emergency room, but this too is a usually compromised version of normal driving, if only in the imperative to go to that place and not to somewhere more pleasant, such as home.

The second—and more common—route is via the emergency medical system. There is not a lot paramedics can do for a patient at the scene of the injury, beyond starting an IV for pain and for fluid replacement and putting a sterile gel blanket over the patient to serve as a heat sink to pull excess heat from tissues. They also secure the patient to a long spine board and immobilize the head with head blocks, thus protecting him or her from further injury. For some patients this care, at least initially, seems comforting, even though this packaging dramatically limits the freedom of the patient. Symbolically, the patient is now "in the system" or "on the conveyor belt," in the slang of the medical world. (Paperwork starts up with the scene-call chart, insurance may be verified, and a chain of referrals begins, from ambulance or helicopter to an emergency room and then to a burn unit.) In theory, patients can always leave the system by refusing treatment, but they are usually in no state of mind to do so.

At the emergency room, the patient stays tied to the board, usually until x-rays have cleared bones for possible fractures. Even after clearance, when straps have been loosened or removed, the patient may be kept on the board, pending transport to a burn unit. Especially after hours on boards, patients often complain about how uncomfortable they are. While there are safety reasons for using boards in this way, a main reason is often the benefit of health-care workers—to limit medico-legal exposure and increase convenience—certainly not patient comfort. Pressure sores, in fact, can result from inappropriate board use, especially for thin and elderly patients. Emergency personnel will cut away clothing (which is then destroyed—unless it must be kept for legal evidence) and cover the patient with a sterile sheet of cloth or paper.

When physicians have assessed the gravity of the wounds and decided that transport to a burn unit would be best, the patient is informed, advised, requested, invited, or even ordered—depending on the training and tact of the treating physician—to travel to the burn unit. If the words are "We need to send you to the burn unit," the patient may feel that the locus of decision-making is external, in the hands of the impersonal and almighty "we." If the words are "Your burns are severe enough that we believe the best treatment for you will be at the burn unit. We'd like you to think about that, ask any questions, talk to your family, and tell us your decision," obviously the patient will feel more empowered and less imprisoned. In some of the most severe cases there may be no conversation at all, since the patient is unconscious, either from the injuries or the attendant shock or from the analgesics (often morphine). The standard of care for such patients is to treat conservatively, which usually means to stabilize them in the E.R. then transport them to a burn center. In such cases the first words a patient hears at the burn center will have strong symbolic import; such words should be chosen with care.

"Where am I?" the patient may moan.

"You're at the hospital. You've had a serious burn, and we are treating it for you." Such a response makes clear that the burn as an event is something separable from the patient—as opposed to saying "You are sick," which is accurate, but has the disadvantage of sounding like the "you" has failed somehow.

Patients arriving at the burn unit by ambulance or helicopter will be immobile on a long spine board. They will have one or more IV lines—the first of many—and may be intubated, which makes speech impossible. They will be on morphine or some other pain-killer. Naked, drugged, and lying on a stainless steel table, these patients are assessed from head to toe and debrided for the first time. Technicians entirely garbed in sterile clothing—caps, masks, gowns, and gloves—pick off dead skin with forceps.

In the intensive care unit, burn patients will certainly have IV lines, a pulse oximeter attached to a finger or toe, and likely a catheter in the bladder; they may be put on a ventilator and will certainly be heavily bandaged. One forearm may be tied to a board to protect the IV site. Drugs keep them immobile. Even vision is restricted: forward and up. In a crowded intensive care room, the view may be only a wall and a ceiling, perhaps medical equipment; only rarely is there a view out a window. Family or friends will look through a glass window to see a person mostly covered up and tethered in alarming ways they have probably never seen. Bulky dressings are designed, in part, to prevent movement, to reduce shearing forces on grafts, for example. They provide protection and conservation of heat, but they also separate the patient from the social world. Family members may have trouble even recognizing a heavily bandaged person (see Figure 8).

Some patients may have "Living Wills," but access to these is often impossible under emergency situations. If the living will prohibits use of emergency measures such as a ventilator, such support may be withdrawn later, especially if family agree. This is a difficult and murky area of bioethics, largely because burn centers are trained to treat aggressively—in the basic rescue model of emergency medicine. It has often been observed that burn-

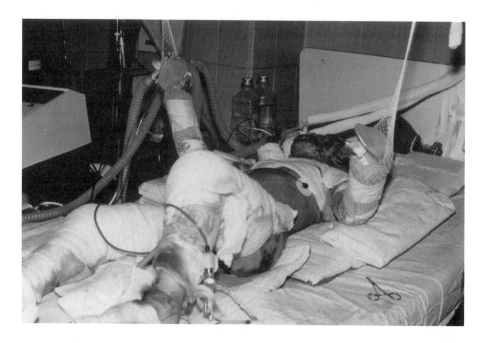

Figure 8. Acute burn. Bulky dressings protect the hands, legs, and upper chest of this patient, all but hiding him. The arm splints immobilize the burned hands, preventing contractures; the netting holds them up to prevent swelling. The patient is on a respirator; tubes and lines monitor blood pressure, oxygen saturation, urine flow, and other functions. Uncovered skin areas and general inactivity make it difficult to stay warm. Photo by Jane Arbuckle Petro.

care workers themselves would not choose to attempt to survive a severe burn, already knowing what is involved, but they treat patients anyway. From long experience burn surgeons usually have a good sense of patients for whom there is no hope, but occasional patients who appear to have been "cooked" to the brink of death make amazing recoveries. Even if patients are given a choice of merely palliative care or a "full-court press," they are often in no mental condition to decide — as are, often, their relatives as well. Another factor already mentioned is the evolution in medical techniques that can now treat burns that were previously regarded as futile to work on. We only signal here some of the conflicting interests about treatment that may suggest yet one more imprisonment, however abstract.

A small child with a burn will be put in a crib (see Figure 9). These often have shiny, vertical metal bars on all four sides — just like bars for an animal cage or a prison window — and sometimes an overhead cover as well. The design of such a "non-climber" is to promote the child's safety, of course, so that he or she won't fall out of bed and risk yet another injury, but the visual

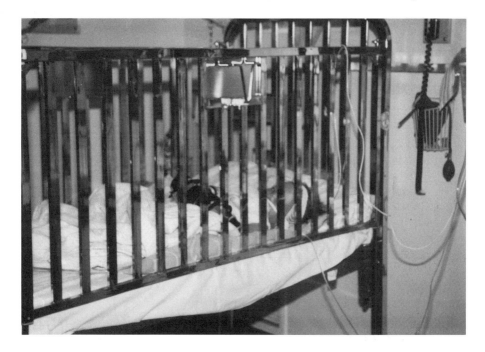

Figure 9. A child's crib. This steel crib has vertical bars so that children cannot climb out. Some have a roof as well, and are used for older children. While safe and easy to clean, such cribs not only resemble prison cells but are in fact imprisoning. Photo by Jane Arbuckle Petro.

effect of such equipment is reminiscent of cages for animals at the circus. A parent will be permitted to spend more time than the usual visiting hours with the child and can raise and lower the sides of this crib, but he or she may still feel that the child is a prisoner in this foreign place.

The geography of the burn unit typically reinforces feelings of isolation. Since their earliest days when infection was a chief cause of mortality, their designs have emphasized remoteness. A burn unit is often hard to find: a distant wing, an upper floor, an out-of-the-way portion of the hospital. There is no entertainment from passersby, no casual drop-ins, no variety of social hustle and bustle, because these sources of stimulation to patients may also bring bacteria, viruses, and molds that healthy people normally tolerate but that may infect and even kill burn patients with their open wounds and in their compromised immunity.

Many patients become dependent on the unit, a kind of "cocooning" or voluntary imprisonment that burn-care workers try to counter. Such patients feel much anxiety about their impending release and whether they can resume anything like normal life "on the outside." Burn workers try to

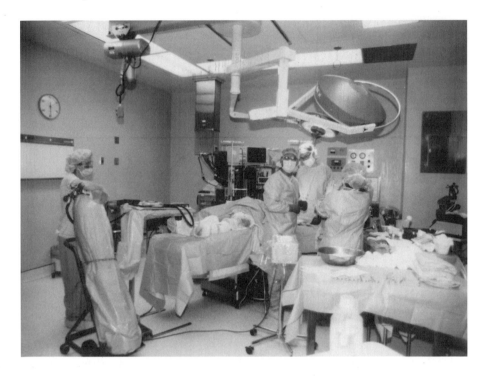

Figure 10. Burn workers. Staff, shown here in an operating room, wear the same coverings when changing patients' dressings: scrub suits, gowns, hair covers, gloves, and often goggles. The patient sees little of them as persons. Even when not in the operating room or doing dressing changes, the staff must wear gowns, gloves, and often masks to reduce the risk of hospital-transmitted infections. Photo by Jane Arbuckle Petro.

make social connections through television, videotapes, even special events in the unit: parties, picnics, even return visits by former patients who can talk about their own transitions. Some more aggressive patients often feel in jail, "out of the way," or "on the shelf." Eager to get back to family, job, social settings, they'll say, "I can hardly wait to get out of this damn place."

Not only is the unit cut off from random traffic, but family and friends find tight controls on visits. The hours are strictly limited, to give staff time for dressing changes and other treatment and to maximize resting time for the patient. A burned man may see his wife just twice a day, for a limited number of minutes, and he will see only a small portion of her, because she will be wearing a disposable gown over her clothes, a cap over her hair, and a surgical mask over her mouth and nose. The purpose of these coverings is, once again, to limit exposure to infection, but they also have the effect of physically blocking off the patient from human communication. All other persons coming into his room — physicians, nurses, technicians, anyone on the burn team — will be similarly garbed. Burn rounds at a teaching hospital may bring a dozen persons into the room, many known to the patients but some (students and visitors) unknown. They stand around the bed in their identical gowns, often with their arms folded over their chests, forming yet another wall in the experience of the patient. It is now common, in the HIV era, for workers to wear eye-shields as well (see Figure 10).

In the unit, life becomes a series of schedules, routines. Dressing changes, rounds, monitorings, administrations of medicine. As the patient becomes more aware of surroundings and pain, pain-killers may become a central focus. Standard of care for pain relief is not by the clock but by relief for the patient — or at least the attempt at relief. Some pain is, despite best efforts, intractable.

Drugs

The use of analgesics is a complicated topic. We will touch on only a few of the imprisoning issues here. The therapeutic aim is, of course, to relieve suffering, and modern drugs are quite efficient. At the same time, however, the patient is often "snowed" to such an extent as to have no awareness, no ability to communicate or otherwise to act like a human being. This twilight existence is particularly hard on visiting family members, who may see the burn patient as a zombie or even, prophetically, a mummy — a wrapped-up dead person. Clearly, burn personnel need to explain how this enforced hibernation is part of the normal healing course. Family and friends may constantly ask, "When will he wake up?" fearing that the answer may be "Never." Such fear may be so strong that the question is not asked at all, a kind of denial. Accordingly, burn workers need to anticipate the question and give the information anyway.

With a conscious patient, another technique, patient controlled analgesia (PCA), has psychological benefits. PCA provides an IV pump within the patient's sight, reach, and manipulation. Naturally there is an overall control (a "block") for the total amount so that the patient cannot overdose, but, within limits, the patient can slow down or speed up the drip of pain medication into the IV line. Both patients and burn workers have seen medical and psychological benefits for patients who feel less imprisoned by controlling their own medication. One of the most troubling issues for patients and caregivers alike is that some pain is intractable: even the most powerful opiates will not block it entirely. In a sense everyone in the burn unit — physician and patient alike — is a prisoner to this physiological-pharmaceutical dilemma. As miraculous as the technology of the burn world may seem, there are some goals it cannot achieve.

The risk of heavy morphine dosage causing depressed breathing is well known, and our society is increasingly facing questions of euthanasia. Currently our society will "put out of their misery" horses, dogs, and other animals, but not humans, even when their injuries are so profound that recovery is either impossible or "unprecedented." This is a difficult area, since burns that were fatal in one decade are often healed in a later time. A well-known article by Imbus and Zawacki, "Autonomy for Burned Patients When Survival Is Unprecedented" (1977), discussed the choice of non-treatment by patients who are likely to die. Nearly two decades later, however, the precedents have all changed and even the gray areas between life and death offer more chance for "bringing patients back." As Petro and Salzburg suggest: "the concept of 'unprecedented survival' changes daily in the burn center" (1992, 616). See also Zawacki on the importance of listening to patients concerning treatment in his editorial, "Tongue-Tied in the Burn Intensive Care Unit" (1989).

The bioethical questions here are complex, of course: killing versus letting die, euthanasia versus murder, active and passive euthanasia, "double effect," and so on. We will simply pose the question: which is the greater imprisonment, a slow dying, perhaps in pain, or a quick death? As of this writing, we have not resolved this issue, although part of Dr. Jack Kevorkian's defense (successful on one case) was that assisting suicide was permissible because he was relieving the suffering of an incurable person who had requested his help. Will this rationale extend to the burn world? Should it? Who can tell when death is inevitable, when there have been some amazing recoveries? These questions will continue to be debated.

Many patients report having no memory whatsoever of their first several days (or even weeks) in the burn unit, and this is surely a beneficent effect, since pain, boredom, and worry are all forgotten. At the same time, we might consider this chemical oblivion an imprisonment of yet another sort, as patients lose a conscious awareness of their own personal history. The body itself has a selective amnesia that protects us from memory of deeply stressful events. While there are some benefits to this forgetting, patients often resent this gap in their memory and repeatedly ask, "What happened to me?" until they can assemble a narrative that is satisfactory to them. The concept of "doctor's orders" may especially rankle; a patient who was formerly highly autonomous may bridle at the control—apparently total—others have over his or her life. According to William Winslade, severely burned patient Dax Cowart saw himself as a prisoner of his physician (in Kliever 1989, 121). While patients have the right to refuse care and caregivers routinely ask for permission to do procedures, patients rarely refuse.

The imprisonments of the burn unit are many, including the state of the burned body, the social isolation, and the enclosing and limiting aspects of medical care. Before turning to psychological and spiritual implications, we'll look briefly at the metaphor of the nursery.

The Burn Unit as Nursery

Because of the helplessness of the severely burned patient, the burn unit has many similarities to the hospital nursery, where infants are fed, warmed, changed, and otherwise nurtured for their eventual departure. Does a severe burn mean that the patient is a baby?

The first answer is "no," since a thirty-year old patient, for example, arrives with thirty years of experience, knowledge, personality, expectations, and so on. Such patients constantly compare their current state in the unit with the life they have typically led. Especially as they make progress toward health and release, they will increasingly resent the limiting nursery-like structures. They or their families may become rebellious, angry. "When are you going to stop treating me like a goddamn baby?" one patient yelled out. What would be the best reply? Perhaps something like this: "I don't consider you a baby at all; you are right now, for better or worse, a burn patient, and my job is to help you get out of this place as soon and as healthy as possible."

There are also patients who recognize the nursery cocoon and come to prefer it to the outside world of stress, choice, and personal responsibility. Some patients regress to a second infancy, accepting their care as a norm, even the best way to exist. Psychotherapy will get some of these patients moving again to reclaim their adulthood. William F. May discusses this rebirth of the burned in religious terms: "The burns . . . destroy the soul's clothing and leave the frail self in naked agony. Then, God willing, the soul begins to grow a new self. The surgeon may be competent to graft skin, but . . . skill alone will not avail to reclothe the soul" (May 1991, 23–24).

Psychological and Spiritual Implications

What are the effects of all these imprisonments? It is hard to generalize, since patients vary, but as patients become aware of their surroundings, they become aware of isolation, profound changes from all their normal life habits, their physical limitations, pain, concern about their accident, and concern about the future. This final circling imprisonment is not spatial, since it includes the patient's perception of all other circles. Even the most ordinary, "well-adjusted" person will feel powerful feelings of depression and/or anger following a major burn. Other patients come to the unit because of previous mental and emotional problems; in a sense, they bring their own prisons with them. "I just love the burn unit," the staff psychiatrist remarked dryly at burn rounds one Monday: "We get so many wackos." Given that he was a gifted therapist of the burned, the remark was not petty vengeance against them, but a sign of his fascination with the varieties of personalities that came under his care. Many patients arrive at the unit with unusual mental states. Some are paranoid; some are drug abusers; some are street people; some have had severe mental and physical problems in the past, which may be the cause of the most recent disaster, the burn.

And then there are stories like this:

> Sam's marriage was on the rocks. While his wife was away at work he sat on her front porch, doused himself with alcohol and ignited the fumes that flowed up his body. His face and chest received especially deep burns.

Sometimes the existing limitations of a patient are not mental but physical, as in the following case:

> Susan was an epileptic whose attacks were usually well controlled by medication. One day, however, her drug level became subtherapeutic, and she had an episode of paralysis. ("Did she stop taking her medication?" asked one nurse.) At the time, she was cooking a meal on a hibachi. As she fell, she upset the hibachi, spilling both the hot coals and the food over her legs. She lay on the ground unable to move for several minutes, sustaining a full thickness burn entirely around both lower legs. At rounds the surgical resident mused—half in jest, half in awe—that this patient had "barbecued herself."

In this case, there were three entities to treat: the wounds, the epilepsy, and the patient's disgust and guilt concerning this macabre event.

As we saw in the Blumenfield and Reddish article subtitled "Small Burn, Big Problem" (1987) some patients arrive at the unit with psychological problems from their past, whether repression of aggressive feelings or complex guilt feelings (to use examples from that discussion). The burn event and subsequent treatment may allow such dilemmas to resurface and to prevent return to a normal life, even when the burn is relatively small.

Death

In Western cultures death is often feared, and many burn patients see in their burns a dread shadow of their mortality. This topic is complex, however, because sometimes death seems attractive.

> A fireman was trapped in a burning building by a fallen staircase, his face shield knocked aside. At that point his rescue seemed impossible, his death certain. In order to shorten his torture, he tried to crane his neck toward the flames so that he could bite the fire and swallow it to bring on death more quickly. He was rescued, however, and taken to the hospital, where he underwent extensive surgery and, post-hospital, a very long period for reconstruction.

Other patients long for death and, finally, achieve it. Sometimes their deaths seem to be hastened by their psychological changes, much like the cliché for dying characters in nineteenth-century British novels: "he turned his face to the wall and died." For them death is no prison. Rather, prison is a life filled with suffering, and death is freedom. Some patients who are religious assume that the afterlife will surpass anything this world has to offer. Said one devout woman: "I don't want any painkillers. My Jesus didn't have any."

There are some other senses of death to consider, besides the usual "final" sense of the term. Many patients are depressed because they mourn the loss of various things in their life: athletic abilities, sexual attractiveness, mental strength to take risks, professional capacities (especially if the burn was work-related), economic losses, even reputation for intelligence and efficiency (especially if they feel that they were at fault in the accident). Such patients may feel that parts of them have already died, that a return to the normal world will never work because they are half-dead: zombies or ghosts, failures or "fuck-ups," returning only in part from the dead.

The case of Dax Cowart became famous after his devastating burn in 1973. His case gained notoriety through the training film already mentioned, *Please Let Me Die*, in which he pleads to be released from the burn unit so that he can go home, become infected, and die. The videotape is disturbing. We watch Cowart, naked and blind, his hands fists of scars, lowered into a Hubbard tank; the water stings the burns all over his body; technicians scrub loose dead skin. The agonized Cowart screams; not only does this particular "tanking" hurt, but it is one of many. In the days when tankings were often used, patients would dread their turn; just hearing the gurney approach their room was an upsetting cue — despite boosts in medicine to dull the pain. When treatment is perceived as continuous torture, surely death is more desirable. (For several perspectives on this case see Kliever 1989.) Dax's case — including his own advocacy — has made possible more patient choice (including refusal of treatments) in the following decades.

Spiritual Aspects

As we have seen in Chapter 1, many of the short books by burn survivors are by persons of religious faith, and all of these profess a deepened sense of the spiritual. (There is undoubtedly self-selection here, since there are also persons who have lost their faith following a severe burn, as well as persons who have an ongoing argument with God about justice — but such survivors tend not to write books.) For some patients the amount of time suddenly available for reflection is a reason for renewed interest in ultimate values, transcendence, and the godhead. Without the hustle of daily routines and chores, even with the hospital television blaring away, patients often ask some version of "What is it all worth?" "What is behind or above it all?" and "Where do I fit in the ultimate scheme of things?" It has often been said that "there are no atheists in fox-holes," suggesting that the mortal threats of war spur soldiers to think about God. The brush with death through a calamitous fire can produce similar reactions for skeptical burn survivors and intensify the spiritual life for those who already have a strong faith. Another factor is the collapse of ordinary, rational structures. Many patients have lived within structures of family, community, work, materialistic gain, and the like; they have prided themselves in having "a full calendar." A sudden trip to the hospital may reveal the arbitrary and ephemeral nature of all of these; if these aren't ultimate values, what are? The answer may be spiritual. Some patients had religious upbringings but grew away from belief in their highly rational and career-oriented 20s and 30s. Sometimes a burn reawakens these earlier beliefs.

The attentions of burn-care personnel and others may demonstrate kindness, love, and grace in dimensions beyond what patients have known (or realized) for many years. A visiting chaplain, minister, or pastoral-care volunteer may give a patient insight into fellowship, spiritual kinship, or blessing. When such a visitor sits at the bedside and listens empathetically, it may be the first time in decades that the patient feels "fully heard," since "everyone is always too busy to really listen." As empathetic as burn-care personnel nurses and physicians may be, they seldom have the time to listen in depth. Sometimes a social worker, a psychiatrist, or even an occupational or physical therapist may have more time to listen and respond. Sometimes family and friends are excellent listeners, especially if they have received information and guidance from the burn staff. Sometimes the best listeners include a minister or rabbi who knows the patient from before, who has seen trauma of many sorts, and who has the trust and faith of the patient.

Sometimes the unit psychiatrist can make a profound contribution to the healing of a patient and his family—even when curing the burn is impossible:

> Leonard was severely burned in a car accident. Horrified neighbors called 911 and tried to extinguish his burning clothes with a garden hose. Paramedics took him to an emergency room, from which he was sent to a burn unit. His wife Sarah, summoned to the unit, found him near death but conscious. The unit psychiatrist observed that Sarah felt not only shock and loss, but anger as well: how could Leonard have done such an awful thing—abandoning her, leaving her a widow with children? The psychiatrist suggested that Sarah tell Leonard all her emotions—sadness, fear of loss, and anger—which she did. She and Leonard talked about her emotions and his, and made up some of their differences. He soon lapsed into unconsciousness. Some hours later, he died.

While Leonard's death caused a tremendous disruption to this family, the intervention of the psychiatrist helped relieve some of the stresses on Leonard and Sarah. Even in the case of a difficult death, the burn unit offered some healing.

Continuing Imprisonments

"A severe burn lasts forever," many survivors say. Here are some of the reasons. Split-thickness skin grafts carry no sweat glands (which lie deeper); these grafts can't cool themselves. With wide expanses of grafts, the survivor doesn't handle heat well, can't exercise in hot conditions. Grafted skin is usually thin and easily injured. It definitely should not be sunburned. Appearances may be altered, especially to the face, even with the best grafting results. People will stare, trying to figure out what's "wrong." A survivor with unusual features — pebbled or shiny skin, asymmetrical features, lost fingers or, very commonly, ears — will receive many stares. He or she will need inner strength to understand these looks and to meet them with verbal formulae. Children stare the most, one survivor found. "Hello," he will say to them. "I was in a big fire, that's why my skin looks like this." He finds that this approach helps the child and helps him too.

Some patients have nightmares about the burn event or the burn agent. Some have phobias about fire, electricity, chemicals — whatever the cause was. Some will not visit the scene again or go to similar places. Some fear barbecues, fires, or life in general, their confidence and sense of reasonable risk gone, burned up, metaphorically speaking, in the fire. Sometimes it's the parents or spouses of survivors who are especially timorous or apprehensive.

In this chapter we have discussed some of the imprisoning senses of burns and their treatment. These provide some of the associational meanings of burns that give burns such a ferocious reputation. In Part III we will discuss how (and to what extent) modern burn care deals with these difficulties. Some survivors gain insight into the limits of the human body and medical care, often gaining a wisdom beyond their chronological ages about imprisonments, mortality, and (sometimes) grace.

Part II
Perceiving Burns Through Images and Stories

Chapter Five
Myths of Fire and Burns

Fire has power that is portrayed through images and stories that are hundreds, even thousands of years old. Some stories show fire's relations with humans and with gods; we have the ancient stories of fire-givers and fire-takers, and animal fables about fire. While many of these have moods of awe and wonder, some — especially those with animals appearing in human-like roles — are humorous. Fire still has fictional roles today, as oral traditions are replaced by film and novels in which fire becomes an agent of change or transformation, often with negative meanings. The phoenix rising from the ashes, reborn into beauty and goodness, today becomes the film character Freddy Krueger (of *Nightmare on Elm Street* fame), returned from the furnace's fire to haunt the dreams of adolescents. Alternatively, the phoenix has become the Phantom of the Opera, who terrorizes virginal sopranos with obsessive love. Fire itself now appears as a sinister character alive and sentient in the film *Backdraft* (see Chapter 6).

Many of the functions of fire, particularly its origins, have been described in myths. We must make clear that the term "myth" means, in this discussion, a symbolic story with explanatory and validating power. For us, myth is a positive and historically accurate term. We are aware that some people interpret myth to mean lie, falsehood, or fairy tale, but that was not the sense of the word in the ancient world. The original Greek word "mythos" meant "story" in all its dimensions: literary, historical, philosophical, and religious (see Eliade and Cassirer). Equally, we may argue that even the most positivistic rationalists of our times live within their own mythological structures, although it would severely pain them to use such a term as myth to represent their own truest and deepest beliefs. In the ancient world, myth was a worthy and useful intersection of religion, cosmology, philosophy, literature, and more — all with the social functions of guiding (and giving meaning to) activities of daily life.

Prehistoric Uses of Fire

While the earliest evidence of human use of fire is somewhat uncertain, archeologists have found burned soil, bones, and stones that were the results of intentional, accidental, or coincidental fires. Finds in Ethiopia, and Kenya dated to 1.5 million years ago contain layers of ash and charcoal that may indicate hearth structures. Deliberate use of fire is first clearly documented in China from the Paleolithic period, about 400,000 years ago: there is evidence of human occupants using fire in the Choukoutein Cave, 37 miles outside of Peking. Contents of this cave include stone tools, split skulls, and animal and human bones, as well as hearths which prove the intentional use of fire (Campbell 1959, 360). The ability to contain fire — to use it for light as well as for heat and cooking — made cave dwelling possible, providing shelter and safe haven even before tool-making and home-making emerged.

Neolithic tools such as drills and flints demonstrate firemaking skills. The ability to make fire must have improved mobility for early peoples since they were no longer tied to specific hearths. The availability of fire was essential for the emergence of tool-making, including clay-baking and wood-working. Fire became a powerful tool for slash-and-burn agriculture, allowing improved productivity for settled populations at least for the short run: such techniques can clear land quickly but with the result that soil is harmed to the point of losing its productive value. Fire's utility in production and destruction required the development, by both nomadic and stable populations, of fire management skill. The emergence of social structures controlling technology coincide with local availability of ore and fuel for burning, initially wood, then charcoal, and more recently coal, oil, and nuclear power.

Humans have always used intellectual structures such as fables, stories, and poems, to define the import and meaning of natural occurrences. Significant events are presented and celebrated in stories with historical, philosophical, and religious dimensions, in short: myths. For example, the Pythagorean view of fire, which arose around 500 B.C.E., was a primary western construct until 1500 C.E. or later. In this tradition, the four elements — earth, air, fire, and water — occur in various proportions in matter and, later, in the four corresponding humors of the body used by Galen to explain the human body and its ills. While this system of only four elements may seem overly simple to us today, it provided a basis for understanding the entire physical world, including human health. This construct provided a rationale for medicine in the west as well as a usable philosophical ideological framework for a much longer period than, say, the modern theory of germs. From its earliest forms, the Pythagorean view had religious and mythic implications beyond the logic of Greek science. Explaining natural phenomena suggests a measure of control over forces that may be physically used but not entirely controlled; typically, all early traditions that we know of have fire myths.

Tales of Fire-Giving and Fire-Taking

Perhaps the most familiar fire-giver in western culture is the Greek figure of Prometheus. According to various Greek versions, Prometheus either snatches fire from the sun or steals it from the workshop hearth of Hephaestus and gives it to humans. Did Prometheus pity humans' coldness and primitive conditions, or did he give them fire and knowledge, aspiring for them to be like the gods? Whatever his motives, he is punished for long ages for his generosity: chained to a rock by the sea, sun-scorched, thirsty, his liver eaten daily by eagles, regenerating at night only to be eaten again. This is a terrible punishment, a hell without fire. With his defiance of Zeus, however, Prometheus is ultimately the victor on behalf of humans: humans, with fire, could challenge the gods — even forget the gods entirely. (In the discussion that follows, we draw some stories from the work of Joseph Campbell and James George Frazer, not because their theories are the last word on culture and narrative, but because the materials they've collected present vividly various aspects of fire and burns.)

According to Joseph Campbell's interpretation of Friedrich Nietzsche, this is the first step in separation from a reliance on religion. The gods are no longer the mighty rulers of the universe but characters in stories, such as those used to instruct and entertain school children in the modern world. Prometheus provides humans the gift that allows them to recreate their own gods, giving humans a spiritual and cultural achievement that usurps their dependence on the pantheon of gods in the old myths and allows a unified interpretation of the natural order (Campbell 1959, 278). In this myth, Prometheus enhances humans' self-perception by lifting them to a role higher than the world of base elements and closer to the lofty dwelling of the gods. Compared to life without fire, the earth with fire becomes like an Olympian palace. The symbolic importance of Prometheus's gift as fire — rather than water, or earth, or air — cannot be overstated. It is fire which most completely allows humans to affect their environment — to heat, light, cook, make tools — all direct outcomes of that gift.

Although a full-scale analysis of the role fire plays in world religions is beyond the scope of this work, a brief survey suggests the wide, even universal fascination with fire and its properties (see *The New Larousse Encyclopedia of Mythology*). Fire is the appropriate symbol of cosmic and epic power. The Assyrians had two fire gods, Gibil and Nusku, who sometimes took the place of Sin and Shamash to dispense justice. For the ancient Greeks, Hestia was one of the Olympians, the hearth goddess; fire was important for cooking and heating, of course, but also as a link to heaven through worship. Hephaestus was the personification of terrestrial fire; his smithy was imagined to be under Mount Etna. He made many things for the gods, including Zeus' thunderbolts and Achilles' wonderful shield (*Iliad*, Book V).

In Slavonic mythology, the sky gave birth to two children, the Sun, and Fire. For the Teutons, the powerful but mischievous Loki is the fire god, and Surt is a fire giant who set the entire earth on fire. This "fatal destiny, the end of the Gods," or Ragnarok, killed both humans and gods, but both were reborn. The Persians had a cult of fire that evolved into Zoroastrianism, and the Vedic Indians had the fire god Agni. Shen Nung, the Chinese deity of medicine, pharmacy and agriculture, was also a fire god. In Japan, Fuji was the goddess of the mountain and also of fire. In America, the Huron and Iroquois believed in a Fire Dragon. In pre-Columbian Mexico, Xiuhecyhtli was a fire god and lord of the sun and the present era. The Incas believed Pachacamac was a god of fire and a son of the sun. In the Pacific isles, stories of the origin of fire are common; variously, it was borrowed, stolen, or a gift, coming either from heaven or the underworld. Parinder's *African Mythology* (1967) lists fire gods and stories for several peoples including the Ila, Dogon, Pygmy, Shoma, Sierra Leone, and Benin cultures. Joseph Campbell, in his *Masks of God* series, presents versions of a number of fire-related myths and tales, some of which we will discuss in a moment. The cumulative power and variety of fire myths demonstrate the significant role fire has played in defining the interactions of humans with their world and the need to present fire in relationship to the most powerful sources of order: gods and goddesses. A few examples will show how fire images in religion reflect the relationship various cultures have had to fire, and through fire, to their gods.

Early Indian Vedic hymns include many songs to Soma (the liquor of sacrifice). Soma is a drink but may also be a god or a king. In one example:

We have drunk Soma; we have become immortal
We have gone to the light; we have found the gods . . . .

Like fire kindled by friction, do inflame me!
Illumine us! Make us rich!
For in the intoxication that you render, O Soma,
I feel rich. Now entering into us, make us really rich as well.
    (Rg Veda III, quoted in Campbell 1962, 181)

Soma was an essential element in Vedic ritual sacrificial practices. These ceremonies, dedicated to and using fire, included chants and actions that allowed communication with the deities, especially those identified with such natural phenomena as wind, water, and fire. Among the most important of these was Agni, god of fire and light, with whom Vedic warriors identified. Their association was symbolized by sunrise, lightning, and the blaze of Agni's fire tongue on their altars. According to Campbell (1962, 180), the altar fires symbolized "confidence in the capacity of aggressive fire to make way everywhere for its own victory over darkness." Soma was poured into the fire as part of the ritual but also into the warrior's gullet, where its purpose was to ignite courage in the warrior's heart.

In the Vedic tradition fully one quarter of the hymns are given to a celebration of the god of battle. Vrita, a handless, footless arch-demon, has hoarded all the waters of the world, leaving the universe a wasteland. Indra, the sun-identified warrior, engages Vrita in battle:

Like a vehement bull, he took to himself the Soma,
Drank the pressed drink from three mighty bowls,
Picked up his weapon, the fiery bolt,
And slew the first-born dragon.
      (Rg Veda I. 32A, verse 3, quoted in Campbell 1962, 182)

The Vedic goddess Indra releases the world from drought with lightning, slaying the serpent / hoarder of all the water. This image of a benevolent deity, one disposed to humanity, contrasts sharply with some aspects of the Semitic god, Yahweh, who uses water to destroy all but a small, selected part of the world, a self-described jealous god who if displeased may become dangerous and vengeful: "For the Lord your God is a devouring fire, a jealous God" (Deut. 4:24). On the other hand, Yahweh guides the Israelites to the promised land with a cloud by day and the fire in the tabernacle by night (Ex. 40:38), which is more popularly rendered as a pillar of cloud by day, a pillar of fire by night.

From this early and very positive image of fire in Vedic culture, we turn to a later and different use, which makes fire a negative symbol of human desire. In the *Fire Sermon*, one thousand years later, Buddha says

All things, O priests, are on fire [. . . .] And with what are they on fire? With the fire of passion, say I, the fire of hatred, infatuation, birth, old age, death, sorrow, lamentation, misery, grief, and despair [. . . .] And perceiving this, O priest, the learned and noble disciple conceives an aversion. . . . And in conceiving this aversion, he becomes divested of passion, and by the absence of passion he becomes free, and when he is free he becomes aware that he is free and he knows that rebirth is exhausted, that he has lived the holy life, that he has done what it behooved him to do, and that he is no more for this world. (Campbell 1962, 210, 212; bracketed ellipses in original)

This later Indian tradition conceives fire and its agent as symbolic of the negative attributes of humanity, an obstacle to be transcended, and calls on its followers to abandon the physical world. The individual warrior and his Soma — the fire-giving drink — are punished, not celebrated. The world has become more complex, good and evil intermingled as elements of each figure in the persona of the gods and in other powerful forces such as fire. The absence of fire, of passion, of inflammation of all sorts is the ultimate transcendence from reality, the truest approach to heaven.

Such shifts in evaluating fire (as well as other evidence) led Campbell— along with James George Frazer in *The Golden Bough*—to group the ancient myths relating to origins into two classes, *myths of the fall* and *myths of the trickster*. The former stories speak of the pride or hubris of humans (e.g., Oedipus) as they attempt to go beyond their natural limits. These stories are conservative in the sense that the universe is ordered by powerful forces that will slap back humans who attempt to rise too high. The Tower of Babel story in Genesis is another example. In the latter group—which includes the Prometheus story already mentioned—the trickster or other hero is a revolutionary figure, a person or animal who dares to challenge the prevailing order, usually for the enhancement of human powers. (We will return to this typology in Chapter 6, when we discuss stories of burns from contemporary popular culture.)

Related tales of fire-giving from early oral traditions have many variants. Sometimes the fire-giver is a simple person or animal, sometimes a trickster who steals and gives fire for no other purpose than the sport of it. One such story comes from a northern British Columbian tribe, the Kaska (Campbell 1959, 277). In this story, fire is held by Bear in the form of a fire stone which he guards jealously. A little bird comes to his den to warm himself. Bear agrees to share the warmth; in exchange the bird agrees to pick lice from Bear's fur. While picking the lice, the bird manages to peck through the string of the pouch holding the fire, snatch the stone, and fly away. Other animals wait outside the den and pass the stone along as each is caught by the pursuing Bear. The stone is finally relayed to Fox, who runs up a high mountain. Bear is so tired he cannot follow. Fox, from the top of the mountain, then breaks up the fire stone and throws a fragment of it to each tribe. And that is why fire is everywhere, in the rocks and in the woods. Folklorists call such tales "pourquoi" tales, those which explain the origins of particular phenomena.

A story similar to the Kaska one comes from the Andamanese tribe from the Bay of Bengal (Campbell 1959, 278). Fire was in the possession of Biliku, a female persona of the Northeast Monsoon, both malignant and benign, the being who fashioned the earth. Kingfisher steals fire from her. When she notices the theft, she hurls a pearl shell at him, cutting off his wings and tail. He swims away and relays fire to another animal, who passes it to the bronze-winged dove. The dove passes it over to all the rest of the animals. Kingfisher, left without a tail or wings, becomes the first human. Biliku, in a rage, flies away to reside somewhere in the sky and never returns.

These tales, of the theft of fire and its deliverance by animals to people indicate both the inter-relationship between human beings and animals, and the superiority of animals and the human need to rely on them. Without fire, humans may not exist (as in the Kingfisher story where humanity comes directly from the fire-thief), or, as in other tales, humans receive the gift from animals, and their life improves. Above all, fire is shown to be magical and worthy of celebration in stories.

Some African tales do not include humans at all. A fable from Sierra Leone is a good example of the pourquoi tale, in this case concerning the leopard's spots (Parinder 1967, 126). This tale explains that Leopard and Fire were good friends, but that only Leopard traveled to visit Fire. When Fire was finally entreated to visit Leopard, a great conflagration ensued from which Leopard and his wife barely escaped. Their bodies have been marked with spots ever since. The story is a cautionary fable: we should be careful what powers we invite into our homes, cities, or cultures at large.

Another African tale has both a spiritual and moral dimension (Courlander and Wolf 1995, 1). This Ethiopian tale tells of a rich man who wagered that his slave could not stand on the top of a mountain for the whole night, naked and without fire. If the slave succeeded he would be made both free and rich. The slave told his friends, who implored him not to attempt it, for he would surely die. Another friend suggested that he might survive if he could only fix his eye on a fire far off, and offered to keep a fire burning on a nearby mountain the whole night. When the time came, the slave went to the mountain top, stood naked, and gazed fixedly at the remote flame. Although he was very cold and suffered greatly, he survived. Others, standing watch over the slave lest he cheat, reported the distant fire to the rich man, who then contended that the slave had indeed cheated and refused to reward him.

The slave was despondent and complained to his friends, who reported this story to other men in the city. One of these men took pity on the poor slave and resolved to help. He arranged to hold a banquet for all his friends, including the slave's owner. On the night of the banquet everyone gathered and sat down to eat. The aromas from the kitchen promised a fine meal, but hours passed and no food appeared. People began to complain until even the slave's owner forgot his manners and began to criticize his host. Said the host, "If the warmth from a fire on a distant mountain is enough to warm a man standing far away, then surely the aroma from my kitchen is enough to be called a good meal." The rich man recognized his mistake and called his slave, granting him his freedom and giving him a large fortune as well.

The key element in this story is the faith of the slave in the power of fire. His ability to warm himself spiritually by the sight of the fire overcame the physical conditions of nudity and the extreme cold of the mountain top. Also important is his faith in the ability of his friend to keep his promise — to maintain the fire — and the demonstration of the inherent morality, if somewhat delayed, of the rich man.

Stories of Hearth and Home

The important relationship between the hearth, or home, and fire can be seen in the tale told among the aboriginal Ainu peoples of Japan. Mt. Fuji, an extinct volcano, is the largest and most revered mountain in Japan. Its sacred nature is not diminished even in modern times by its popularity as a mountain-climbing goal and tourist destination. It is named for the fire goddess Fuji, who was the ancestor of the Ainu people and the goddess of the hunt (Campbell 1959, 335–41). According to the Ainu tradition, when a wild bear is killed in the mountains it must be brought into the house of the hunter through an opening known as a "god's window." The mountain goddess, knowing that the bear has come to the house, also comes down from the mountain to share in the feast. The bear is set next to the hearth where, for twenty-four hours, it converses with Fuji, who is both the goddess of the mountain and the goddess of the hearth. The bear and the goddess share memories of their common home, the mountain. After this, the bear may be skinned, cooked, and eaten, and the goddess enjoined to return to the mountain.

The ancient Greeks also had a hearth goddess, Hestia. This link between the hearth, fire, and a goddess is common to many cultures, providing a link between femaleness, fire, hearth, home, heat, cooking, and nourishment. Such figures are called "laric" after the Roman "Lares," guardian spirits — usually female — of the home.

Fire in the Bible

The listings for "burn" and "fire" in Strong's *Concordance* are considerable (*Burns, Burned, Burneth, Burning,* and *Burnt* account for over 800 references; *Fire* for some 600). Without detailed commentary, we list a few of the more vivid uses. "Then the Lord rained down on Sodom and Gomorrah brimstone and fire from the Lord out of heaven" (Gen. 19: 24). God speaks from a burning bush which does not consume: "And the Angel of the Lord appeared to him in a flame of fire out of the midst of a bush: and he looked, and lo, the bush was burning, and yet it was not consumed" (Ex. 3: 2). "Mt. Sinai was wrapt in smoke, because the Lord descended on it in fire" (Ex. 19: 18) and again, "Now the appearance of the glory of the Lord was like a devouring fire on the top of the mountain in the sight of the people of Israel" (Ex. 24: 17). Other references include various offerings burned on the altar and fire and smoke in worship. In the New Testament, fire descends as the Holy Spirit at Pentecost (Acts 2: 1–4).

God also uses flames to reveal innocence. In the Book of Daniel, King Nebuchadnezzar orders a furnace to be heated seven times more than usual in order to destroy three of his subjects who will not worship his gods. When Shadrach, Meshach, and Abednego are cast into the "fiery furnace," an angel of the Lord leads them through the flames unharmed, to safety. Here God rescues these loyal worshipers, protecting them from the pain and annihilation of the most intense flames available to the King.

In Numbers (21: 4–9) the Lord sends fiery serpents to bite and kill the people of Israel. This chastening by the Lord is tempered when the Lord instructs Moses to "Make a fiery serpent, and set it on a pole; and every one who is bitten, when he sees it, shall live." So Moses made a serpent out of bronze and put it on a pole. This symbol, along with the staff and snake of Aesculapius (adopted son of Apollo, another healer) is a forerunner of emblems for medicine today. (This symbolism, however, became confused by the American military symbol of the double snakes on a winged staff, the caduceus, which was originally the wand of Hermes/Mercury, a trickster messenger. Strictly speaking, the most accurate medical image would be a staff with the single snake, as seen on many hospitals, rescue units, etc.) In many ancient cultures, the snake carried special symbolic powers for healing and resurrection because of its ability to shed its skin and to appear rejuvenated, as if reborn directly from Mother Earth.

In some ancient stories the flames are helpful or even redemptive, while in others the flames are punitive — this latter sense informs the medieval imagery of hellfire and damnation and the burning of witches.

Burning Witches, Electrocuting Criminals

Early Christians endured persecution that included burning, as illustrated by Saint Lawrence on his bed of fire. Later, the church itself used a stake and fire to punish suspected witches, especially heretics. The death of Joan of Arc in 1431 may be the most famous such burning. Although she was called a witch, it was as a heretic that she was burned. Her disruption of the social order was both political and military (Williams and Adelman 1978, 29–32; Ginzburg 1991, 97, 100). Her "heresy" was as much her challenge to the established political order as her religious claims.

The event also shows a complexity of values attributed to fire. Her persecutors could not lose: if she was truly a saint, the flames would not harm her and she would be spared; then her tortures would be praise-worthy for showing her true power. After all, stories of many saints showed their imperviousness to pain: Lawrence, when grilled over flames, called out to be turned over in order to cook the other side. If Joan was a fraud, however, she would perish in the flames, an appropriately tortured scapegoat whose death would serve as a lesson. (This strategy worked equally well with the ducking stools in colonial America.) Joan's death was, therefore, a proclamation of her guilt, and a victory for the clerics and military leaders who condemned her. By this consciousness, fire is capable of proving the existence of good in the world, or of punishing and expunging an evil force.

Later, witches were burned, drowned, or hanged. Even more recently, electricity (a modern equivalent of fire) was developed as a supposedly more humane means of capital punishment, even though the descriptions of the first uses of the electric chair are gruesome. An early electrocution in America used too much voltage and caused the head of the victim to burst into flames. A. Conan Doyle, observing this new technique from afar (England), was moved to write a tall-tale account, "The Los Amigos Fiasco," in which too much electricity extends the life of the criminal instead of killing him (1894).

Hellfire and Damnation

The earliest images of hell, sheol, or the underworld were not dominated by fire, with the possible exception of the Hebrews' Gehenna (or garbage dump), although some passages in 2 Enoch have fire imagery, according to Alice Turner (1993, 40, 49). Turner also suggests that a reference in Isaiah (14: 9–15) refers ironically to hell, using Babylonian imagery. Otherwise, the Hebrew Bible is relatively devoid of images of any afterlife. The concept of a fiery punitive afterlife is largely a medieval construct.

Plato gave the mythic realm of Hades detailed structural form and reality in his *Phaedo* and *The Republic* (Book 10). In brief, the platonic theory of forms suggested that worldly corporeal existence is a degraded form of the ideal reality, so that a "pure" existence in the afterlife must exist, reached only after death. When Socrates considers his own impending death, he reassures his companions that there is, indeed, such an afterlife. The soul itself is an ideal form which is eternal. With good behavior in this life, it will pass to Hades, a desirable destination for the deserving. The wicked, by contrast, are punished by reincarnation back into the corporeal or imperfect world.

By the Middle Ages in Europe, hell had a well defined landscape dominated by fire (except in Icelandic traditions where hell is ice) and an accepted role in church doctrine. Dante, for example, used both fire and ice imagery in his *Inferno*. This concept of hell as a place of punishment, especially through fire, had a popular hold on the imagination of the masses, most of whom could not read Dante, but who could see portrayals of flames and the shrieking damned in mosaics, bas-relief sculpture, and other art. (Dante himself saw such mosaics in his neighborhood church in Florence, now the Baptistry of Santa Maria del Fiore.) Sermons, both in Latin and increasingly in the vernacular languages of Europe, further spread the hellfire and damnation imagery and doctrine. Such sermons continued through the colonial preacher Jonathan Edwards ("Sinners in the Hands of an Angry God") to James Joyce's *Portrait of the Artist as a Young Man* (the interminable Chapter 3) and Steve Martin's movie *Leap of Faith*, as well as other images in fundamentalist preaching.

There are, of course, other uses of fire. In the New Testament, for example, the fiery tongues of the Holy Spirit that reach listeners of all cultures at Pentecost. Fire is sometimes a refining or cleansing element, sometimes an indication of God's presence, even in haloes or other imagery of illumination.

There are many other traditions of fire that directly or indirectly shape our attitudes toward fire and its threats to us. In the Norse tale of Brunhild, Odin punishes her by putting her to sleep, surrounded by a ring of fire. Here fire is a barrier, a protection, and a test. Siegfried must ride through this ring to win Brunhild. Both in the original Norse myth and in Wagner's late-romantic operas, fire is seen as magical and moral, combining love and death, and capable of eliciting from humanity its most heroic and triumphant aspects.

How do these images of hell, fire, punishment and damnation affect the patients in a burn center? It is hard to imagine anything more hellish that the burn injury itself and the pain associated with lengthy treatments of burns. Indeed, patients familiar with stories of hellfire and damnation frequently understand their burns to be an infernal punishment, surely for some evils or crimes they have committed. Even caregivers who also carry similar images from childhood stories and religious training may see themselves as participating in a hell on earth; are they devils administering punishment, or angels providing comfort? Perhaps burn workers—burn-care providers and fire-fighters as well—are, mythically speaking, heroic Siegfrieds, riding through the flames to rescue a beloved person. Or maybe the burn patient is Siegfried-like, in helping to create his or her own rescue. Such mythical imagery may help us understand the conflicts which patients and their caregivers feel during and after hospitalization, not just for burns but for any painful condition.

Overlaps of Christian and Non-Christian Myths

The ceremonial use of fire on many occasions reminds us that we are not as far from dependency on fire as we might think. What follows are descriptions of some of the more modern uses of fire in symbolic ritual. (Our source for many examples is Frazer's *Golden Bough* 1922.)

Christian ceremonies have always incorporated and adapted elements from the cultures around them. In Europe the practice of Lenten and Easter fires combine mid-winter fertility rites with the beginning of Lent and the related spring celebrations of the Easter renewal. Frazer describes communal fires set on peaks about the town, fire brands carried through fields and orchards, and ashes applied to hens' nests, fields, and orchards—all to insure fertility. Newlyweds would leap over the flames, and unmarried youths would seek luck from the fire. The burning of effigies, variously called witches, Old Man, or Old Woman, was also common, especially in the Easter fires. Death, resurrection, and fertility combined to bring a good harvest.

According to Frazer, the roots of effigies — magical substitutes for persons or animals — go back at least to Roman times, possibly including Celtic and druidical practices. In some cases the victims were not substitutes but actual victims, such as condemned criminals who were burned — along with various animals — in large cages. Modern-day burning of persons in effigy or flags of nations or even brassieres all are strange survivors of these events. Other versions include self-immolation, usually for political and religious purposes, which we discussed in Chapter 3.

Beltane fires were lit on the first of May throughout Wales, England, and Scotland. This practice lasted well into the nineteenth century, and persists or is being revived today. In origin these fires were brush and wood set aflame on high hills to chase away evil spirits, especially those believed to affect milk and egg production. Cakes and custards made of milk and eggs were baked and eaten, and in some rituals those accused of crimes were challenged and threatened with burning. In many places all other fires were extinguished before the Beltane or the Easter fire and then rekindled from the main fire later. This practice recalls rituals requiring the general extinction of all fires and their rekindling when a new king is to be crowned, or the Vedic ceremonies to Agni, the fire god, rekindling all fires annually from the "tongue of Agni," the altar flame. Some Christian liturgies use a similar distribution of candle-lighting from a central flame.

Midsummer's eve and Halloween are additional festivals of fire. Halloween, incorporated into the Christian year as the eve of All Saints Day, marked the return of the souls of the departed and the release of devils who could move freely on that night. Fires lit on that night served to prevent the influence of such spirits and to provide omens for the future. Modern children go from house to house at Halloween with flashlights powered by electric batteries, while jack o'lanterns (perhaps with an actual candle, but often with a light bulb) glow from windows and porches.

The midwinter fire ceremonies, coinciding with the winter solstice, have been incorporated into Christmas celebrations via the Yule log. Yule logs per se are rare today, but fires in fireplaces are not, and Christmas tree lights (electric versions of the Victorian candles on trees), along with indoor and outdoor lights on houses are common in the United States and elsewhere.

Large, community directed ritual fires exist in modern times as well. The Louisiana Cajuns along the river between New Orleans and Baton Rouge hold a Christmas tradition of building elaborate, enormous log towers which are then ignited on Christmas Eve. These towers are evenly spaced along the river bank, each proudly identified by the family that built it, in annual competition for biggest, and best (*New York Times* 24 Dec. 1995,

p. 10). This tradition goes back at least 200 years and has an uncertain origin. The purpose may be to light the way of the faithful to church for Christmas Eve mass, or to welcome Papa Noel, or both.

Regularly scheduled ceremonial fires have often been augmented by special fires, called "need-fires." These were used in medieval times at times of distress or calamity, for example, an epidemic, especially one afflicting cows and other animals. Such need-fires have two meanings. One is the symbolic, the purifying force of fire, can be seen as having creative and destructive potentials, as it consumes bad influences or chases them away. The other is the relationship to the sun and the seasons, especially the returning spring and summer of fertility and life.

This brief review of the wide range of legendary and mythic materials on fire suggests the broad symbolic power fire possesses, representing human hopes and fears. Fire cleanses and destroys, creates and punishes, gives hope or terror, provides public and private spectacles. This polarity of fire continues to find expression in modern interpretations of ancient stories. We will now turn more specifically to two such ancient myths that influence our contemporary perceptions of burns: the stories of Icarus and of the phoenix.

Icarus and Phoenix

In our reading, these two stories represent contrasting interpretations of disasters in general, fire-injuries in particular. In Chapter 9 we will apply these stories to the reality of burns and modernize them to reinterpret the meanings of burn injury.

The story of Daedalus and Icarus is known in many versions, but perhaps the fullest is in Ovid's *Metamorphoses*. In this version, Daedalus, a fabulous craftsman, is held prisoner on the island of Crete by King Minos. Minos has exacted technological service from him, having him build the labyrinth for the Minotaur (itself a product of another of his constructs, a mechanical heifer in which Queen Pasiphae could hide in order to copulate with a bull). Daedalus plans with his son Icarus to escape on wings he has constructed out of feathers and wax. On the day of the escape, the sun burns brightly. Icarus ignores his father's warnings about the fragile wings and, intoxicated by the power of flight, soars too high toward the sun, causing the wax to melt and the wings to disintegrate. He falls to his death while his helpless father watches. Various artists and writers have retold this tragic story, including the poet W. H. Auden ("In the Musée of Beaux Arts") and the painter Pieter Breughel the Elder (*Icarus*). By his invention Daedalus is in the tradition of the "fall" narratives of fire, although it is not he but his son who falls, both physically through space and psychologically through the seduction of a godlike power.

The story has entered our culture with all its mythic power as a kind of icon or norm. *If you misuse technology, you will suffer.* (Other versions include the Tower of Babel, Dr. Frankenstein and his monster, and the Sorcerer's Apprentice, made available to thousands of viewers through Walt Disney's film, *Fantasia.*) The fall of Icarus is a result of high spirits and lack of temperance; it is a brutal punishment, a deterministic trajectory. The Breughel painting shows his tiny white legs disappearing into the sea while a boat sails by and a farmer plows on, both unheedful of the tragedy near them. This story, we contend, has become a subconscious model for disasters in general and burns in particular. Its message is that such falls are inevitable, deterministic, and fatal. *Too much technology will get you into trouble; fly too close to the sun and you'll get your wings burned and die.* Furthermore, *no one will care.* The story may even be read as a normative myth for contemporary humanity and technology. *Unless we change our attitudes and behaviors, we shall all die because of our obsessions with materialism, energy in all its forms, and depletion of natural resources; we will be doomed to crash and burn in an Icarian, ecological disaster.*

In contrast to the pessimism and fatalism of the Icarus story is the story of the phoenix, the mystical bird that dies in a fire only to be reborn from an egg found in the ashes of that fire. In brief, the phoenix is an image of hope, optimism, and infinite creativity. The phoenix story has many versions — Persian, Chinese, Egyptian (the benu bird; see Figure 11), and Roman — and variants with other creatures: scarabs, snakes, and butterflies, some of which we've already mentioned. Humans have a fascination for symbols of ways life may be extended or regained, whether through animals, fountains of youth, or acts of gods. (Tithonus was made immortal, but he forgot to ask for youth to go along with his never-ending life.) Mediterranean gods who exemplify a death-and-new-life paradigm include Tammuz, Osiris, Orpheus, and, of course, Jesus of Nazareth. Indeed early Christian readers interpreted a Latin poem "The Phoenix" by Lactantius as an allegory for Jesus' death and resurrection. This poem may have been the source for an Old English poem, also called "The Phoenix," in which Jesus and the phoenix are made explicitly parallel.

The bird is an especially suggestive image to humans because of its freedom to fly and — in the case of the phoenix, to roost at the top of a tall palm tree. In the Roman version (Ovid's *Metamorphoses*), the bird lives 500 years, then builds a nest of sweet spices in a tall palm tree and dies amid this fragrance. A baby phoenix arises from the nest; gaining strength, it carries the nest (a tomb for the old bird but a cradle for the young one) to the city of the Sun (Heliopolis) and lays it at an altar, an offering to the sun-god. In this recounting there is no explicit story of burning, but a clear reference to the all-powerful sun, the source of all heat and all life. The story, in general, is quite positive in its values of renewal and celebration.

The Greek historian Herodotus gives a similar version in his *History*, but this hard-headed rationalist casts doubt on the tale, which he finds fantastic

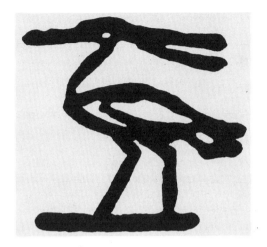

Figure 11. The Benu bird. This hieroglyph shows the Egyptian version of the phoenix, the benu (or "bennu") bird. We like the English pun on "be new." Image adapted from *The Egyptian Book of the Dead.*

and incredible. In fact the story gives hints about how the dead were actually prepared in Egypt, using herbs and chemicals. Specifically, the body of the phoenix is so treated, then entirely wrapped up like a mummy to await its rebirth. (Among burn patients and their visitors, perhaps the elaborate bandages suggest a mummy-like preservation and a cocoon from which new life will spring.)

The image of the phoenix has stayed alive in many forms. The city of Phoenix, Arizona owes its name to founder Darell Duppa, who noticed remains of canals and villages from the earlier Hohokam civilization at the site and determined that the new city would rise from the ashes of the old. Basil Spence, an architect, described the rebuilding of England's Coventry Cathedral, bombed by the Germans in World War II, in his book *Phoenix at Coventry* (1962). Edward D. McDonald edited papers of D. H. Lawrence, whose reputation was then at a low ebb and entitled the volume *Phoenix* (1923). Burr Cartwright Brundage wrote of the mesoamerican figure Quetzalcoatl in *The Phoenix of the Western World: Quetzalcoatl and the Sky Religion* (1976). Clearly the concept is alive, well, and still evocative to many.

An opposite to the Icarus story, the phoenix story offers perfect renewal after a fire, and even makes the fire a pleasant, celebratory, and life-preserving event. Alan Jeffry Breslau, founder of the Phoenix Society of Burn Survivors, speaks of the phoenix rising from the ashes "more beautiful than before." As an ideal, the phoenix story gives the most positive version possible, one that can give burn survivors hope and enhanced self image. This story symbolizes an extreme of hope and positive envisioning of burns, much as the Icarus story symbolizes the opposite extreme of negativity and despair. Both stories tell us a lot about the range of human desires and perceptions, and it is important to have both. The Icarus story functions as a cautionary tale, a warning to humans not to endanger themselves, while the phoenix story functions as a story of inspiration and hope, urging humans to see beyond tragedy and death.

Even today, fireplaces typically add to the value of a house, even though they often have no practical worth since they send heat right up the chimney. Bonfires still play important ritual roles in adolescent life (high school and college pep rallies), and summer camps and wilderness programs often use campfires for values far beyond mere cooking. Lighting candles for birthdays, for many religious rituals, and for romantic dinners—all these further attest to fire's symbolic role and some of the positive and enabling myths, now largely forgotten but central of the experience of many persons in the past and throughout human history. At the same time, we have stories of burning witches and effigies, even the destruction of entire evil cities, as well as modern news accounts of fatal fires, the Holocaust of World War II, the images of Hiroshima, Nagasaki, and a final "all-out nuclear exchange." All these relate to stories of the end of the world in flames, various versions of the Apocalypse. Myths describe the deepest meanings and values of fire; they show—whether through folk tale, scripture, or film—the wide range of responses and interpretations humans have created about fire. A burn survivor may have a powerful mythic reservoir informing her or his experience; these influences may be helpful or not, encouraging or not, clarifying or confusing. We believe the Icarus and phoenix stories influence the deepest (and often unexamined) assumptions of burn patients and of burn-care providers.

The figures and stories we have reviewed in this chapter attest to the power fire has held in the human imagination. Through millennia, as boon and bane, as friend and foe, present at the origin and the end of the world—fire holds unique, magical, and evocative power over us. To stand next to fire, especially for persons not in the modern industrial age, has been akin to standing next to a god. For a burn victim, a sudden physical encounter with fire may be an experience of sublime terror. The meanings attributed to the inchoate experience of a severe burn will depend on the mythic models, conscious or not, that live in the minds of patients, their extended family and friends, and the medical community which assumes responsibility for the survival and recovery of the burned.

Chapter Six
Darkman and Other Images of Burns in Popular Culture

In this chapter we will look at contemporary stories that provide, for better or worse, evaluative and moral meanings to fire and to burn injuries. Movies, comic books, and novels, we find, contain some of the clearest and most influential representations of social values, many of which derive from the myths just discussed. One vivid example is the movie *Darkman* (1990), which portrays a renegade scientist trying to make artificial skin. When his lab is blown up by thugs, he is horribly burned, then miraculously healed by a heartless physician who uses him as a guinea pig. He escapes the hospital to continue his own scientific research and to plan revenge on the villains who maimed him and delayed his work. We see several of the themes and images of the Crane story "The Monster" here, including the ingenious scientist who works beyond limits that society can comprehend. Both stories are tragic in the tradition of the "fall" narratives we saw in Chapter 5. Many of the other exhibits we have chosen to use here, including the "super-hero" comic books, also show the modern fallen world. The super-heroes, virtuous in themselves, labor continuously against the injustices and super-villains of the world. Such villains are usually conveniently marked, often by burn or acid scars (as in the Joker), stigmata that signify evil within. Within these narratives, the villains often challenge the powers of the universe. They work their schemes for personal benefit or, occasionally, for the benefits of others. They may fail, ultimately, as do Dr. Frankenstein and the Joker, but the effects of their actions often live on, as in the promethean gift of fire or the Joker's criminal empire.

Popular Culture: Reflector of Values, Guide to Values

The power of the mass media is hard to over-estimate, given the saturation of television, film, radio, and print media. An example of an image that reflected and created values is Nick Ut's "Napalm Girl," a photograph taken

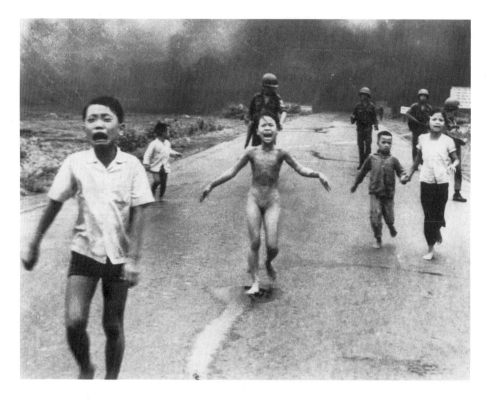

Figure 12. "Napalm girl" by Huynh Cont ("Nick") Ut, June 8, 1972. This often-repeated photograph of children fleeing napalm became a pivotal image for the American conscience as people lost enthusiasm for the war in Vietnam. AP/Wide World Photos, used by permission.

in 1973; the following year it won a Pulitzer Prize (see Figure 12). Widely circulated, this photograph showed several children fleeing an accidental napalm strike. At the center is a nine-year old girl running down a country road, naked, with her arms outstretched, face distorted with terror and pain. She has lost her burning clothes and runs toward us, as if begging for our help and protection. "Napalm Girl," more than twenty years later, still remains one of the defining images of the Vietnam War.

This image dramatically portrayed the impact of the war on non-combatants, a concept that had been reported in print media for some years but never with the force of this photo. The image Ut projected contrasted sharply with government reports of statistics, including "kill ratios." Americans reading newspapers at home suddenly saw a personal example, an "identified life" in the bioethicist's phrase, of children suffering, *victims* as sacrificial offerings for some religious purpose. Here the religion could only

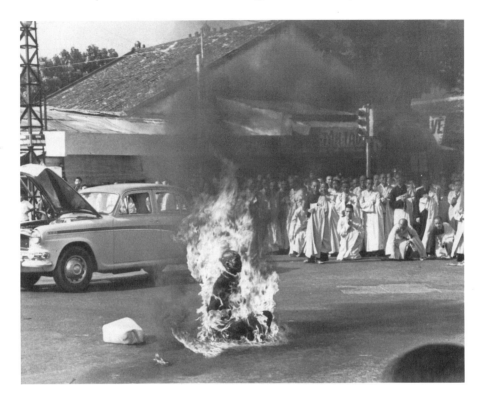

Figure 13. Self-immolation for social protest, Saigon, Vietnam, June 11, 1963. Quang Duc, a Buddhist monk, doused himself with gasoline before thousands of onlookers to protest alleged persecution of Buddhists by the Vietnamese government. AP / Wide World Photos, used by permission.

be seen as a pointless war, and this widely disseminated photograph has been credited as one of the major influences in the shift of American attitudes about that war. Ut's photograph redefined what American weapons of fire were doing "over there."

After taking his monumental photograph, Ut rushed the girl and her brother to a Vietnamese hospital, where she spent 14 months in recovery. American plastic surgeons did much of the skin grafting required to treat the burns that covered 50 percent of her body. Today, Kim Phuc lives in Toronto with her family. In 1996 she laid a wreath at the Vietnam Veterans Memorial in Washington, D.C. (*St. Petersburg Times*, 12 November 1996, A-1, A-8).

Other vivid portrayals of fire that influenced public opinion about the Vietnam war were the photos of self-immolation by Buddhist and European antiwar activists (see Figure 13). A new image of the burn victim emerged, that of hero and moral protester. The photograph we have chosen shows a protest against the government of Vietnam for its repression of Buddhist monks. Photographs of such deaths were widely published, and their dramatic effect stimulated the discussion of what was appropriate or not for TV news. The U.S. government especially did not approve of the images being portrayed. It is impossible to ignore images such as this one, to look away, to avoid the enormity of the subject matter. Clearly the conflagration is final, complete, and permanent. Once again, instead of numbers or distant images of a town burning, we have the isolated figure of a human being in an intense relationship with fire, a relationship that is dramatic, rhetorically powerful, and, of course, fatal.

Pain and Deformity in Mass Media Entertainment

In a culture that is both pain aversive and obsessed with physical beauty, the mass media epitomize, in their stylized fashion, the ways we look at pain and deformity. Since the primary goal of mass media is the creation of profit, however, the images of pain and deformity are heavily interpreted — even explained away. While the pain of the real life "napalm girl" is clear enough, the pain of cartoon characters is often hidden or suppressed entirely. Wily Coyote in the *Roadrunner* cartoons, for example, is never hurt, no matter how many times he falls off a cliff, is blown apart, or is flattened by a heavy object. There is a long tradition of pain-free characters such as St. Lawrence. In contemporary stories, by contrast, a character who does not feel pain is often a villain, for example, Dr. Doom, an evil scientist burned in a lab explosion. We know that the ability to feel pain is a basic part of being human and a point for empathy between a fictional character and ourselves. Absence of the ability to feel pain implies deep deficiencies in physiology, character, and morality. The experimental treatment employed by the doctor in *Darkman* involved the elimination of pain sensations in the brain, resulting in a significant change in behavior as well as perception.

Deformity is another marker that we interpret variously. On the one hand we have the tradition that external deformity must mean internal deformity of character, as in the Joker, Freddy Krueger, or the Phantom of the Opera. On the other hand, a marked character may be sympathetic, a kind of an ugly duckling who represents the insecurities of reader and viewers whose own looks may seem inadequate or incomplete. Examples include Cyrano de Bergerac, in either Rostand's late-romantic play or Steve Martin's movie version (*Roxanne*, 1987) and the clubfooted hero of Maugham's *Of Human Bondage* (1915). In each case they are defined, at least in part, by their deformity, even while they aspire to transcend it. Perhaps at root for both pain and deformity is the basic dilemma we have with evil in a culture that no longer has a unifying mythology, a theodicy that makes sense of the world's limitations and injustices. Or we could make a slightly different point, that the dominant ethos of the upper classes includes such invariable beliefs in progress, in economic justice for those who work hard, and in the generally predictable and orderly nature of the world, that it does not include — let alone explain — personal tragedies, especially if the tragedy is absurd, unaccountable, or unjust. While we lack a clear understanding of evil, we are nonetheless eager to know about it — fascinated even — and thus ever vulnerable to the images and stories of the mass media.

The Trickster and the Limits of Technology

In stories of the trickster, the central figure challenges the powers of the universe, whether divine or mundane, using wits and an innate sense of play as well as ambition to create wider powers. This theme combines well with the vivid and dramatic powers of fire, as seen in such movies as *Phantom of the Opera, Batman, Darkman,* and *Nightmare on Elm Street,* and in the characters who are transformed by fire, such as Darkman and Freddy Krueger. Here the trickster, like Prometheus, acts as an intermediary for higher powers and transmits gifts to others, such as fire, power, health, good luck, or even bad luck. A still more speculative point is this: that technology itself may be a trickster, offering ever larger powers only to withdraw them or to taint them with dangerous shortcomings. Prime examples include Dr. Frankenstein's "life sciences" and the Sorcerer's apprentice's magic. For fire and burns, the argument could run like this: modern humans are so entranced with energy that they deplete the world's resources, burn a hole in the protective ozone layer, pollute air, water, and earth, and superheat their world to the extent that human life will no longer be possible at previous levels of comfort and safety. From this perspective, burns are just one marker of our ambition, greed, and carelessness.

Mass Media and the Meanings of Burns

What is the meaning of being burned and surviving in our society? This question will dominate much of this chapter, and the answers we offer are many. Such answers are important for the unburned, as well as those who have been burned or who are otherwise involved in the burn world. Answers derive from the larger meanings of fire in both historic and mythic terms, and from our contemporary alienation from the realities of fire. Ordinarily, contact with burn survivors is unusual and in-depth familiarity rare. While death and destruction by fire are frequently major news stories, we tend to perceive such news as disasters that happen to *other* people, entirely remote from our own domestic experience with fire. Thus when personal burns occur, they are a shocking intrusion, unexpected and unreal.

In our analysis, a severe burn as shown by mass media presents a variety of unclear and conflicting meanings. It can be: (1) a punisher of evil, or a sign of intelligence; (2) a form of purification or a tool of torture; (3) a gift of the gods, or God, or an attribute of Satan; (4) a symbol of the end of the world; or (5) the burning of a city's trash, be it in the literal or figurative sense, as in burning our street people in their own campfires or electrocuting convicted criminals. Since the visual properties of fire convert very well to cinematic images, film-makers take advantage of our confusion to impress us with explosions that threaten both heroes and villains on the screen (*Speed*, *Blown Away*, *Die Hard*). Since film-makers know how vulnerable our instincts and imaginations are to fire, they use them heavily for dramatic, thematic, and climactic effects. In turn, these products influence our perceptions of fire and burn survivors.

In the following discussion, we will look at *The Phantom of the Opera*, *Darkman*, *Nightmare on Elm Street* (with its endless set of sequels), and *Backdraft*, focusing on how fire and burns are presented and interpreted by this powerful medium. Film, the graphic medium by which we are commonly entertained and educated, and whose images help define the times in which they are created, has replaced the newspaper serial and many of the popular live arts, such as traveling theater shows and burlesque. Despite predictions that TV will rule, films still attract huge audiences, reflect popular tastes, and influence much of popular culture — as well as eventually filling air space on TV. After our discussion of films we will also look at some modern novels' treatment of burn injury and deformity to explore whether literature reflects the values seen in the films.

The Phantom of the Opera and Other Masked Faces

In no other modern story do we have our ambivalent feelings about the burn survivor and our unconscious feelings about burns and disfigurement revealed as repeatedly and as clearly as in *The Phantom of the Opera*. The original French novel, written in 1911 by Gaston Leroux, tells a story of a congenitally deformed genius who falls in love with a chorus girl and helps shape her career and engineer her fame by acting as a kind of Machiavellian Pygmalion. In the end he wins her love, only to be rejected when she sees his deformed face. When the mask is removed, his revealed deformity demonstrates the enormity of his evil and the basic immorality of his character. In the novel, this deformity is a congenital condition, not a set of burn scars. The Phantom's deformity was life-long, not the result of life-changing burns — which the films introduced for ready-made symbolism.

Phantom is the only one of Leroux's fictions to survive in popular culture, although during his life it was not his most successful work. A popular novel, it was translated into English and German and it sold briskly as both a book and a newspaper serial. Its popularity for later generations was ensured, however, when it was first made into a film in 1925. The story subsequently gained a life of its own, having been filmed repeatedly, and recently (1994) running in three separate theatrical stage versions. The transformation of the Phantom from congenitally deformed to burned is a clue to the fascination that this story has on the modern imagination.

While visiting Paris in 1922, Carl Laemmle, president of Universal Pictures, met Gaston Leroux, who, in addition to being a novelist was also a film producer. When Laemmle shared his excitement over the dramatic size and style of the Paris Opera House, Leroux gave Laemmle a copy of his novel. Laemmle read the novel entirely that night, and decided to produce the film in Hollywood and use Lon Chaney as the Phantom. Universal already had a Paris set, made for its production of *Hunchback of Notre Dame*, which also starred Chaney. Chaney, known for his genius at makeup and his ability to portray monsters in a sympathetic and sensitive manner, created a Phantom who was evil and frightening, but also touching and pitiable.

This first *Phantom of the Opera* film was released in 1925. A silent film, it used wild gestures, over-dramatization, and dialogue cards to convey the Phantom's inner nature and depth of feeling. Christine, the young singer, takes voice lessons from the Phantom, who keeps himself hidden behind a mirror (another symbolic touch). When she sees him for the first time, the card reads, "Look not upon my mask — think rather of my devotion which has brought you song." The film explains that his injuries resulted from torture during the French Revolution; thus the iconography of villainy attains another dimension: evil stems in part from the evil of his torturer. The first film does not dwell on the specific mechanism of the Phantom's disfigurement, but the image revealed when he is unmasked at the end is a face covered with the taught, shiny skin of a burn survivor and the upturned nostrils and staring eyes that can result from burn-scar contractures (see Figure 14).

Other images that arose from the first *Phantom* film include the mask, the black flowing cape, and the broad-brimmed hat that have become conventions for the evil genius (including Darkman) as well as for the romantic rogue (Zorro, the Phantom of the comic strips, Batman). Produced just before the advent of sound in films, this version remains the most powerful rendering of the dramatic relationship between the Phantom's character and his face. In 1930, with sound now available, Universal reengineered the silent *Phantom*, adding music and dialogue, and re-released it in that same year. Despite modern preferences for sound, the original version, without dialogue and score added, is the better film.

The theme of the Phantom has been repeated in subsequent films with several gradual transformations: first, unequivocally into a burn survivor (an explanation that survives in subsequent versions) and then into a completely unsympathetic, evil being. The theatrical version, a musical by Andrew Lloyd Webber, restores some of the sympathetic qualities of the Lon Chaney version, but the essential fate of the Phantom remains that he cannot win the girl, and that he must die.

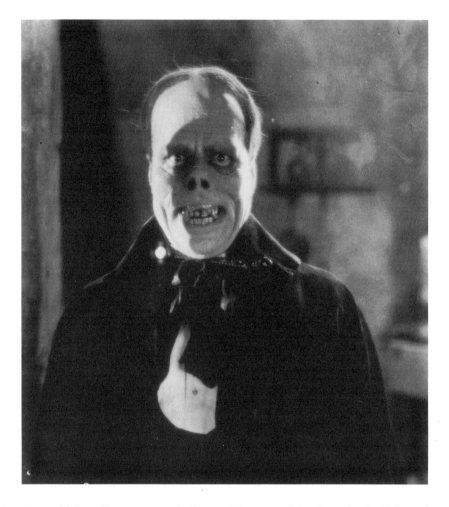

Figure 14. Lon Chaney, unmasked, as the Phantom of the Opera in the Universal Studios 1925 silent film. *Phantom of the Opera* publicity still.

Appendix 1 provides a brief overview of the many Phantoms of the past fifty years, demonstrating the continuing fascination and economic value the character has had in contemporary popular culture. The films show a wide range of variations—some quite ingenious—that films take from previous versions. Such extensive use of the story illustrates the assumption by film-makers that audiences yearn to see rituals of harm and horror. These films, with their conventional images of innocence oppressed by cruel and evil experience, demonstrate such evil through symbolized burn imagery. Evidently this assumption holds up in practice—even in some of the worst versions — since viewers have avidly consumed almost all these versions of the Phantom. Although absolute proof would be hard to assemble, we believe that these many and pervasive images are influential in maintaining and intensifying social attitudes of disgust, revulsion, and rejection of burn survivors. At the same time, we see the human impulses for excitement and danger in encountering extremity as well as the curiosity to know about these fascinating but different people — even if they are to be reductively interpreted and rejected.

The genre of popular horror films in the 1970s and '80s often featured burn survivors as agents of mass murder and terror. Jason, resurrected from the dead by lightning in the *Friday the Thirteenth* series, and Freddy Krueger in *Nightmare on Elm Street*, were not, however, normal (let alone innocent) when they were burned. Freddy Krueger, in particular, is guilty of a most horrible crime, child molestation. The town's people seek to exterminate him in the tradition of burning witches by throwing him into a furnace, but his supernatural evil transcends even this extreme punishment — a demonic reversal of the biblical story of Shadrach, Meschach, and Abednego. Symbolically, Freddy's burning transforms his evil from the material world to a supernatural dimension from which he can return to haunt and kill in the dreams of the children of his murderers. The premise, that dreams can be real and dangerous, coupled with the degree of mayhem committed by the terrifying figure of Freddy, made this apparently interminable series of films major box office successes among adolescent audiences, who have purchased versions of his mask and knife-like hands for Halloween costumes. One critic, in a review of *Nightmare on Elm Street 5: Dream Child*, referred to Freddy as "America's best loved knife wielding burn victim." His makeup exaggerates burn scars, contractures, and still open wounds to a grotesque degree never seen in clinical medicine (see Figure 15).

Cult classics such as *Texas Chain Saw Massacre* and the terrible *Friday the Thirteenth* films likewise feature severely disfigured burn survivors. Somewhat less grotesque is the burn disfigurement of the character the Joker, played by Jack Nicholson in the first *Batman* film. These film images universally ascribe an evil nature in direct proportion to the facial disfigurement of the burn victim. Such images, it is safe to say, are a powerful influence on our response to actual burn survivors, especially among children but even among adults, regardless of how much we profess to be free of bias.

The modern variations of masked evil, in the slasher/horror genre, shows burn injury in a less complex manner than in the Phantom tradition. Many horror films of the 1980s used the masked figure as a simple icon of evil, dehumanizing the character and turning horror into a simple matter of multiple brutal murders. Repetitive sequels to *Halloween*, *Texas Chainsaw Massacre*, and *Friday the Thirteenth* stimulated numerous discussions of the decline of the film industry and the loss of creativity among not only makers of the films but consumers as well. The chief benefit of these films seemed to

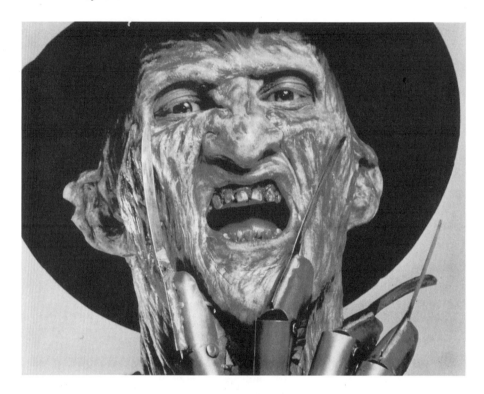

Figure 15. Robert Englund as Freddy Krueger—possibly the most common (not to mention repulsive) image of how Hollywood distorts a burn survivor's appearance. The appearance resulting from the elaborate makeup bears little resemblance to that of a healed survivor, even without modern treatment. The only possibly correct detail is the undamaged eyes; wonderful reflexes almost always spare eyes from flame. *Nightmare on Elm Street*, publicity still.

be the revenues each subsequent version could generate. Whether such films have contributed to increased violence in society—and especially violence against women—has also been debated widely. Politicians have used the possible impact of such images as a justification for attempting to impose censorship.

Darkman

In our opinion, the best version of *The Phantom of the Opera* since 1925 is the 1990 film *Darkman*. The Phantom in this case is a scientist researching mechanisms for remaking faces with artificial skin. Burned in a laboratory arson fire, this Phantom is shown as a patient in a burn center—a rarity in film—but with a fantastic and wildly inaccurate visually dramatic presentation. He is being treated by a woman surgeon (another rarity) in the Dr. Frankenstein tradition; she uses him, an unidentified burn survivor, as a guinea pig. Her experiments to control pain in burn patients include damaging certain centers of the brain. She tells a visiting group of scientists that the one negative effect is the loss of control of feelings. Darkman is her captive, bound on a machine that is a grotesque combination of Stryker frame, wheel of fortune, and crucifix (Figure 16). Upon hearing her describe her experiments, Darkman breaks his bonds and leaps out the window (apparently several stories up), escaping to find and exact revenge on those who burned him. What makes this particular film different and better from the usual B-movie is the care given to developing the character of the scientist Darkman. His attempt to rebuild his lab and continue the search for an effective artificial skin, his search for redemption and revenge, his acknowledgment of his lost self, his mourning the loss of his girlfriend — all coupled with images reminiscent of earlier scientists/monsters/phantoms — combine to give the film sympathy, intelligence, and effectiveness. The black cape and broad brimmed hat, masked features, intelligence, and longing for love all link him with the other Phantoms (see Figure 17). Film buffs enjoy knowing that Liam Neeson, who plays Darkman largely under wraps, later played the highly visible Schindler of *Schindler's List*.

Three stage versions of *Phantom of the Opera* were in production in the 1980s and '90s; two of them show different esthetic and thematic aims. The Andrew Lloyd Webber musical, enjoying a long production run on Broadway (among the ten top all-time money makers and longest running shows), was preceded by Ken Hill's production, mounted in 1984 at the Royal Theater, Stratford upon Avon. Hill presented as a camp version of the original *Phantom of the Opera* story, a combination *Rocky Horror Picture Show* and West End musical. Lloyd Webber saw the Hill play but could not conceive the dramatic structure until he found a used copy of Leroux's novel in a bookstall and realized the romantic potential of the story line. The Lloyd Webber theatrical version — while remaining true to the novel in the murder and deception practiced by the Phantom — does not contain any of the horror of the novel or the silent film version. Instead, the Phantom is highly romanticized and portrayed as a sympathetic character who longs not to be evil but is somehow compelled by his deformity to act as he does. In the conclusion, love does redeem him, although it cannot save him.

Thus the Phantom has been slowly transformed, evolving through many versions from a complex character to an almost cartoon-like figure of evil, until rescued by the romantic and sympathetic character of the Lloyd Webber musical. The 1911 novel gave him a life history and a development. He was congenitally deformed but also brilliant, participating in the design and building of the Paris Opera House, where he could take up his shadowy residence. His lifelong animosity, clearly derived from his experience, requires no sudden, inexplicable character transformation. Later Phantoms, burned

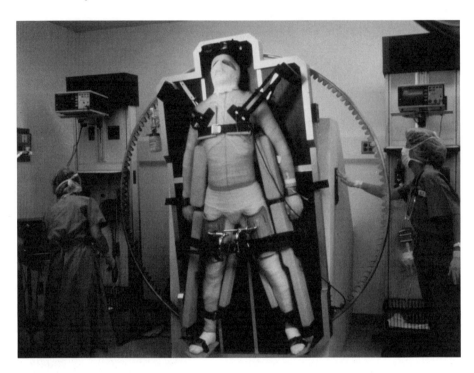

Figure 16. Darkman as a burn patient. This somewhat exaggerated contraption is a combination of several systems used to protect (restrain) and turn patients. It is not like anything commonly used for burn care but seems to combine a wheel of fortune, a crucifix, and an orthopedic bed called a Stryker frame. On the other hand, the mummy-like bandages around Darkman's head and neck and the compression garment on his chest and arms are familiar sights in the burn center. *Darkman*, publicity still.

in mid-life or later, are somehow transformed by that burn into wicked persons, mechanically losing humanity. The symbolism of burn deformities representing lost moral values links the Phantom story to the witch-burning of medieval times: those who are untouched by fire are clearly good and can escape punishment; those who are marked by fire are clearly bad. One attraction of the Phantom story, therefore, lies in its ability to rationalize evil, to create a simple justification for its existence, and to show how, once humanity is lost, even love cannot restore the Phantom to his original self. The unjust nature of the burn injury, inflicted on the Phantom by some intrinsically evil minor character (in some versions an impresario, a music publisher, etc.) suggests that even innocence can be corrupted and that goodness is not necessarily a salvation or a state of permanent grace.

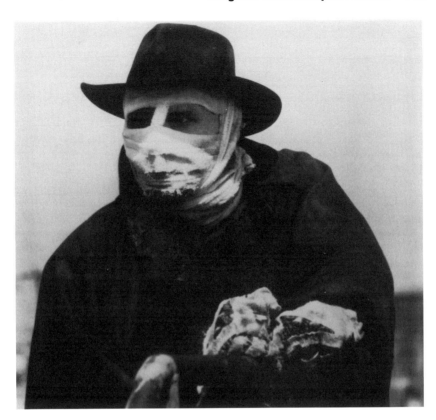

Figure 17. Darkman, a variation of the Phantom. The unkempt bandages, black hat, and cape are hallmarks of the burn victim as horror hero. *Darkman*, publicity still.

The modern conversion of musician into scientist and opera house into research laboratory, and the commentary on the uses and misuses of medical science, also suggest transformations in the roles music and science play in society. Technology, as friend and foe, Frankenstein as man and monster, and ultimately the inability of technology to reverse fate leave Darkman trapped in his transformed self. As he says in rejecting his girlfriend's offer of continued love and assistance, "I am not the same man I was. I am changed on the inside by what I have become on the outside." The unconscious message is that a severe burn and its treatment can profoundly change an ordinary person into a vengeful monster of uncanny powers, a scapegoat that we should all reject. When Darkman blends into the crowd at the end of the movie, we have the thrill of knowing he is still among us. So also, we may presume, is the irresponsible doctor who changed his psyche while providing "medical care." The inevitable sequel to this film, *Darkman II*, is best avoided.

Super Heroes and Super Villains: The Perils of Radiation

Another set of contemporary popular culture images that shape our response to disfigurement is the super hero comic book. In this mass medium, characters are intensified and simplified, as either super heroes or super villains. There is little variety in the origin of the powers associated with these characters; the usual source is exposure to some form of radiation, a decidedly modern (and particularly frightening) form of burn. What distinguishes the individuals as good or evil is the presence or absence of disfigurements. Super heroes don a disguise to hide their human, normal selves. Super villains, on the other hand, assume various disguises either to enhance their disfigurements to frighten others or to disguise their nearly inhuman appearance.

Young adolescent and even adult collectors of super hero comic books avidly purchase Spiderman, Batman, Fantastic Four, and Superman comics in quantities of hundreds of thousands per month. Widely read, exchanged, and collected, these comics are an important source of culture for their fans. Young readers, with their evolving minds and sensibilities, are fascinated by relationships between evil and disfigurement and by the attractiveness of truly good characters. The Fantastic Four, in particular, have been enormously popular: four teenagers, who through their special gifts and magical transformations are able to combat evil, while not frightening people around them. Such traits appeal especially to anxious and awkward teenagers. The Fantastic Four are built on the ancient four elements, including fire, the basis for the Human Torch.

Converting popular comic heroes into TV and film stories has recently brought a resurgence of interest in these figures, starting with *Superman* and more recently *Batman*. The disfigurement of Batman's opponents in the comics has been translated to the screen with two prominently burned characters, the aforementioned Joker of the first film of the series, and Harry "Two-Faced" Dent in the third film. Like that of the Joker, Harry's disfigurement is a result of acid burns—which he blames on Batman. Harry's dual nature, a split personality of good and evil, is reflected in his physical appearance, one side handsome, the other scarred and twisted from the burn. The other opponent in the film, the Riddler, was transformed from a techno-nerd to an evil trickster by the rejection of his ideas by Batman's alter-ego, Bruce Wayne. Thus both characters are *created* evils, seeking revenge on their change agent.

For our purposes, the continued representation of evil by a burned figure challenges us to consider whether these injuries influence burn survivors' acceptance back into society. The disturbing implication—in comics, in film, and (as we shall see) in literature—is that moral nature is directly reflected by physical appearance, and that transformation of character, from good to evil, may be externally caused by the experience of injury. The role of popular culture in articulating contemporary fears and beliefs is not new or unusual. Our current obsession with beauty—an attractive "acceptable" appearance—and the frequency with which cosmetic surgery is discussed, recommended, and used seem to complement the symbolism of deformity to show moral failing.

Inarticulate concerns about nuclear matters, the "bomb shelter" mentality of the Cold War, and the recently revealed extent of experimentation done on unwitting and unconsenting human subjects are all part of the background for the B-grade monster movies of the 1950s. The vague concerns of that decade were exploited by films; later, such concerns turned out to have validity. In 1994, when the Energy Department of the Clinton administration began to solicit complaints from those possibly exposed to radiation in the 1950s, they assumed that three "hot lines" would serve to field the not more than 100 calls predicted. Within two weeks the service was receiving 500 calls an hour (Lee 1994).

Movies from the 1950s—especially B-grade mutant movies—frequently used radiation as a harmful force. The 1954 *Them*, about giant ants evolving from common insects after radiation exposure, 1955 *Tarantula*, on a similar theme, and the 1957 *Amazing Colossal Man*, the story of an army colonel—all portrayed exposure of government misdeeds, careless handling of dangerous materials, and cover-up efforts designed to keep the truth from the public. The 1990s government revelations about the nature and extent of the experimentation done in the 1950s (information released by the Energy Department under the guidance of Secretary Hazel O'Leary) confirms some of the suspicions of such popular culture, even though it seemed to have little merit in its day.

Fire as Sentient Being

Fire itself plays an important role in comic books and film. It is used as a weapon, as a key to survival, or even as an identity: the "Flame" and the "Torch" in the comics referred to in the previous section. It is also the causative force in transformations, as we have argued, occurring in explosions of nuclear materials, chemicals, electricity, or other flammable substances. Fire can also be a character, used as an anthropomorphic figure in, for example, *Bambi*, *Backdraft*, *Towering Inferno*, and *Carrie*. If we watch a fire spread in a room (see Appendix 2 to this volume for a description of fire behavior) we may have the impression that it has intelligence as well as momentum: first moving slowly, gradually gaining strength and potency, moving faster, becoming hotter and hungrier, pouring out smoke to obscure its progress until it leaps up in a rage to consume all the contents of a room or an entire building, radiating enough heat to crack windows and melt distant objects. Such fires are used in *Towering Inferno*, in *Bambi* (fire disrupts the natural world and frightens audiences of children), and in *Carrie* (fire springs directly from the body of an adolescent girl, a symbol for her rage). Cinematographers love fire for its symbolic, dramatic, and, of course, visual qualities. Even a bad movie will often end with a spectacular fire scene, as if the director hopes, somehow, to pull off something in a frantic blaze or explosion of glory (*Zabriskie Point*, 1969).

Backdraft (1991) is a special-effects extravaganza that capitalizes on the sentience of fire. This film is about arson, murder, filial rivalry, and the Chicago fire department. The murders are combined with arson, using a phenomenon known as "backdraft," the sudden introduction of oxygen-laden air to an enclosed space so that a small, smoldering fire explodes violently into flame. Robert DeNiro plays a fire investigator teaching one of the rival brothers how to detect arson. His slightly sinister character is revealed in a long shot of him changing his shirt with his back to the camera to show burn scars. In one of the most memorable scenes, DeNiro's character starts a fire at an investigation site and shows a young fireman how fire progresses and moves around and across a door frame, all the while murmuring to the flames, "talk to me, tell me, talk to me." In this film fire is not simply a special effect; it is a malevolent and intentional character. The climax, a chase scene in a burning, chemically toxic building, presents one of the best visualizations of fire and fire fighting ever seen in a movie.

The use of fire as a character in film—with the excitement and drama that fire lends to the cinema—has spawned a small growth industry of special effects. From the short, singular yet powerful explosion at the end of *Zabriskie Point*, the use of special effects has become a dominant force in films like *Backdraft*, *Speed*, *Blown Away*, and the *Die Hard* series. Early film fires, as in *The House of Wax*, *Frankenstein*, and *The Bees*, were means to a moral end, the destruction of the evil place. In these more recent creations, the fire is generative as well as destructive, more alive, and vital to moving the plot forward, not signifying a resolution. This romantization of fire ignores the daily reality of the toll fires take in the destruction of property— residences, businesses, and forests—and perhaps reflects our alienation from fire as a powerful force.

Spontaneous Human Combustion

This phenomenon, headlined in the tabloid press (*National Enquirer*, *World Weekly News*, *Star*) proposes that human flesh can spontaneously ignite and completely burn away, occasionally leaving behind a foot or part of a shoe. It was a well described fiction even in the nineteenth century; for example, Charles Dickens in *Bleak House* (1852–53) ascribed the death of the drunk,

Mr. Krook, to "spontaneous combustion." Philosophers and scientists of the day decried Dickens's promotion of the popular misconception, accusing him of perpetrating "a vulgar superstition" and "complete ignorance of all the causes or conditions which preceded the accident and caused it" (Nickell and Fischer 1986, 353).

The dramatic image of such spontaneous combustion (for example, "Preacher Bursts into Flame Giving Hellfire Sermon") suits the style of the tabloids, but overlooks the effects of fabric ignition and prolonged burning of flesh which more rationally explain the mysterious deaths of Dr. J. Irving Bently or Mary Reeser, frequently cited cases of alleged spontaneous human combustion. Bently, a famous St. Petersburg, Florida case, has been particularly kept alive in the oral tradition; more generally, the popularity of spontaneous combustion as a folk motif can be seen in its regular appearance in the press since the early 1800s (Blizin, Krogman, Nickell, and Allen). The readiness with which readers and even "responsible" media (Blizin) believe in such accounts indicates a fascination or fantasy or even faith in fire far out of proportion to its natural capacities. In reality, the combination of intoxication with smoking is responsible for most of the cases proposed as spontaneous combustions, as well as the majority of fatal house fires in the United States. Some materials such as damp hay can "spontaneously combust" (even this language is somewhat misleading) when processes of natural decomposition accumulate enough heat for ignition — but not human flesh. Still, something in the popular mind wants to entertain such extremity as a mysterious possibility.

In a twist on the theme of spontaneous human combustion, films like *Carrie* or *Firestarter* capitalize on the possibility that thoughts can initiate fires. Portrayed in both films as emanating from adolescent females, this ability symbolizes the emergent sexual power and instability attributed to young girls. In these movies repressive (and repressed) adults who attempt to control such girls instead experience their power and are incinerated; no wonder adolescents enjoy such films.

Some Novels of Fire and Burn Survivors

A number of contemporary novels also use fire as a character. Like the movies, these works tend to interpret burn-related facial disfigurement to deformity and evil or to profound personal unhappiness. A few novels are described here as examples and do not represent a comprehensive or even representative exploration of the theme. Nor does this discussion seek to evaluate the relative artistic value of these works. They represent a range of artistic effort from contemporary popular fiction through works of aesthetic seriousness. The common motif is burn deformity as a mark of character, a stigmatizing, dramatizing force, implacable and inescapable.

During the 1950s an extremely popular genre of cheap adult novels could be found in the racks of urban drug stores. They had titles like *It Rhymes with Lust*, *Wild Town*, *Shana and the Lost Tribe*, and *Swamp Kill*. The covers, in color, typically showed a woman wearing provocative clothing, in a suggestive pose with flames behind or actively consuming her, but strangely untouched. These bold images link fire with sex, sin, and lust. Surprisingly enough, these novels were widely available during the McCarthy era, publicly displayed, and very successful — despite the era's television image as a model time (*Leave it to Beaver*, *The Nelsons*, or that "wacky but lovable" Lucy). Furthermore, there was nearly always a lesbian love theme graphically depicted in the text. Fire, flames, sex, sin, and taboos all melded together narratively and graphically in a fifties version of pulp fiction, the penny dreadfuls of the post World War II era.

Jonathan Kellerman's psychological detective story *Private Eyes* (1992) illustrates the compelling desire of the facially scarred to escape stares. A once famous movie actress, now a recluse, has developed agoraphobia following an assault with acid. The scars, after many operations, are actually slight, but the result is unsatisfactory to the actress, who is visually obsessed and perhaps vain. The conclusion of this mystery both identifies the reason behind the original assault and resolves her psychological distress enough that she is able to go out again. Although such a resolution and healing are medically plausible, they are rarely found in fictional treatments, which tend, especially in detective fiction, to follow the "looks bad means is bad" formula, for example in Joseph Stanford's *Eyes of Prey* (1991).

Another example of the burn survivor as a sympathetic figure (also a woman) is the Hartford Circus survivor in Mary-Ann Tirone Smith's *Masters of Illusion* (1994). Tirone Smith's work of historical fiction is a fascinating account of the life of one of the survivors of the real-life Hartford Circus disaster and her husband's obsession with the cause of the fire. He is — appropriately enough — a firefighter. The book is rich with descriptions of the circus fire, firefighting, and the slow process of finding and interviewing witnesses, participants, and others many years after the event. Tirone Smith uses the Hartford Circus fire as the dramatic cause for mystery-solving to understand both the events that started the fire and the dilemmas of the characters. Fire is similarly used in the 1979 French mystery, the prize-winning (Grand Prix de la Littérature Policière) *Trap for Cinderella* written pseudonymously by Jean-Baptiste Rossi. Two young women are burned beyond recognition in a resort fire; one dies, but the other is saved and reconstructed into a beauty through plastic surgery. Who is she? The rich or the poor one? The murderer or the intended victim?

Fire dominates the opening scenes of William Golding's *Darkness Visible* (1979). In this novel Golding continues his exploration of human character and the relationship between moral values and opportunity. In *Lord of the Flies* he recreates the chaos and cruelty of modern society out of the "innocent" band of adolescent youths abandoned on a desert island. *Darkness*

Visible begins with firemen battling a blitz-related fire in London during World War II. We have already described the kinds of fires that are incompatible with life — backdraft and flashover (the total ignition of a volume of space). A young child, Matty, emerges from just such a blaze, his presence so startling that the first firemen to see him are unable to move to rescue him. Matty emerges from the fire to seek an identity beyond merely being a burned person: "the question which went with him always, changed and came clearer, Not — *Who* am I? *What* am I?" This question later changes to "*What am I for?*" In the end, the novel is unsatisfactory; though filled with beautiful writing, it never answers these compelling questions. The figure of Matty remains trapped in his body, ashamed of his face, unable to make meaningful human connections. He is, in short, an image of the burn survivor as a highly limited person, especially in psychological and social dimensions.

Kobo Abe's dramatic Japanese novel *The Face of Another* (1966), is an extended meditation on the meaning of faces and masks. A chemist, burned in a lab accident by acid, unexpectedly comes to realize his own vanity and his inability to cope with his lost face, which symbolically stands for his lost identity. Using his chemical knowledge (parallel to that of Darkman), he begins to make a mask for himself, becoming convinced that it is realistic and effective. Initially he says, "No matter how many faces I have, there is no changing the fact that I am me" (19). He continues to experiment with his mask, and while doing so begins to move about in the town with his bandages still on. While sitting in a railroad station he considers: "I wondered if I weren't becoming a kind of monster. Carlyle said that the robe makes the priest and the uniform the soldier; perhaps the face makes the monster. A monster's face brings loneliness, and the loneliness informs his heart. If the temperature of my freezing loneliness were to drop even slightly, I should become a monster, indifferent to my appearance, and break with a crash all the bonds which bind me to this world" (61).

Once again, the external wound changes the psyche. When the mask is complete, it satisfies him and enables him to break out of loneliness and reconnect to his wife and colleagues, only to find out that the mask is seen just as a mask, and that only he is fooled into seeing it as a face. This realization is devastating. Even with his external appearance normal and acceptable to the public, he knows that he has changed within: he has fully become criminal. Accordingly, he puts on the mask for the last time and goes out to commit random murder in order to cross the line *in action* from man to monster. Abe shows us, dramatically and insightfully, that the loss of a face, especially the loss through burns, creates a terrible burden for the survivor. A mask may conceal, but it cannot reconstruct a lost identity. (This novel was made into a black and white film *Face of Another* in 1966, produced in Japan.)

Golding and Abe both show the sorrow, mourning, and suffering of the survivor, but these authors provide neither positive insights nor solutions for survivors or for the non-burned who encounter scarred people. Nor do they take any easy or conventional routes to excuse responses to the face or to invent a convenient, warm person with special power (someone blind, perhaps) to see beyond the face. The face is gone. The person is lost. And, as in many films, that loss leads to cruelty, to disregard, to some form of evil.

Keiji Nakazawa's *Barefoot Gen: The Day After* uses a comic book format to follow one boy, Gen, through the horror of the aftermath of Hiroshima. The line drawings of the dead and dying and the survivors of the bomb are as pathos-filled as any photograph could render. As Gen searches for his family, his search becomes a metaphor for the search for humanity in an inhumane and terrible world. It is a moving work of art, story-telling, and political testimony, which — despite the cartoon format — deals realistically with the impacts of radiation burns on a large scale.

First-Person, Non-Fiction Accounts

We have discussed works of fiction, theater, and film; in the previous chapter we looked at myth and fable — all in relation to fire. We should not leave out first-person accounts of catastrophic events, since these can show dramatic physical aspects of fires and, of course, the psychological impact of these fires on individuals and cities at large. There are also powerful indirect accounts such as John Hersey's *Hiroshima* (1948) or Norman Maclean's *Young Men and Fire* (1992), which relives the terror of forest fires. Images of people, cities, and fire — whether the great fire of London (1660), Chicago (1871), Dresden (1945), or Hiroshima (1945), provoke terror and awe.

The Great Chicago Fire of October 8, 1871 illustrates some of the fire science, social attitudes, and human responses to adversity that are central to this book. Since, furthermore, it has been very well documented we will give more attention to it than we have some of the fiction described so far. Five years before the Chicago fire, the Fourth of July fire (of 1866) in Portland, Maine, destroyed half the city and provided the first use of documentary photography in recording a non-military urban disaster. The dramatic images and well documented fire fighting techniques employed in that fire contributed to the adoption in many cities of fire fighting improvements. (The costs associated with insurance losses had caused the collapse of Portland in 1775 when the British burned it to the ground; in another touch of irony, the Casco bank, which had burned down previously, had chosen the phoenix as its symbol.) The fire in Portland resulted from a combination of factors, including a hot dry summer, high wind, inadequate water supply, and an origin in the waterfront section of the city where the lumber mill, molasses factory, and other wooden buildings provided efficient fuel. Impacts of this fire included changes in the architecture of the city (from Federalist to Victorian), widened and straightened streets, and the enact-

ment and enforcement of a rigid building code (Ryder 1983). Similar results occurred in New Orleans (French colonial to Spanish-style), and in
San Francisco, Baltimore, and Chicago.

The origin of the Chicago fire, the notorious (and documented)
O'Leary's barn, was truly at the heart of the fledgling city, although the
villainous cow and incendiary lantern are best characterized as elements of
folklore. In 1871 Chicago was a city of over 300,000 people, bordering Lake
Michigan in an area six miles long and three miles wide. It had developed
from a village of fewer than 100 inhabitants organized and named Chicago
in 1833. The village was built on the site of Fort Dearborn, which had been
wiped out in an Indian attack during the War of 1812. Like the fort, a
trading post on the frontiers, Chicago was a city of commerce, its business
and wealth deriving from its geographical location: its position on the great
lake provided a natural pathway to the West. Chicago continued to be a
major port even as the railroads began to replace water transportation.
Shipping, trade, and manufacturing supported the booming economy. The
location of the city was, however, problematic for construction. It was built
on a marsh, with the result that mud was a major hindrance to building
streets and sidewalks. The most readily available building materials came
from the great northern pine forests of Michigan and Wisconsin. Thus, although some brick, stone, and iron construction occurred during the rapid
expansion and building of Chicago, most of the buildings were pine, as
were — surprisingly enough — the street curbs and sidewalks. Furthermore,
to reduce mud exposure, the sidewalks were elevated, some as high as 6 or 8
feet. This height ensured that they would be dry and open to wind from
below, and therefore readily combustible.

The fire danger to Chicago was well known. In 1858 the city had consoli-
dated its once numerous volunteer fire departments into a paid, professional department. The professional firemen were well regarded and well
paid, and — because of the frequency of fires in the wood-built city — well
experienced. Their equipment was modern for that time, including horse
drawn steam pumps ("steamers"), twelve in all, and a water delivery system
throughout the city that included hydrants at regular locations. The city
water supply was ample and well powered with a recently completed water
station drawing fresh lake water from intake valves two miles out in Lake
Michigan. Chicago did not burn because it was unprepared.

The summer of 1871 was dry. Less than five inches of rain had fallen in the
preceding three months. Trees had already shed their leaves. The sidewalks
were like dried kindling. The fire department was overworked and a number of its members were ill, injured, or exhausted. During the weekend of
the Great Fire numerous smaller and one major fire had already been successfully controlled. The entire department had been called out on Saturday night to help extinguish a fire that had started in a planing mill on the
southwest side of town. Before it could be contained, the fire had consumed

four city blocks. It has taken 16 hours to control the fire and the department had lost several pieces of equipment and was running out of fire hose.

No one knows for sure exactly how the catastrophic fire started, although newspaper accounts reported that Mrs. O'Leary's cow had kicked over a lantern in her barn. The cow has since been considered innocent. Nor was it "divine retribution for the burning of Atlanta by Sherman's troops" as claimed by the Rushville (Indiana) paper, the *Democrat*. The fire did, however, start about 8:45 P.M. in the O'Leary barn at 137 De Koven Street, not far from the preceding night's lumber yard fire. A delay in sending the general alarm, plus the central fire tower's mistaken impression that the glow in the neighborhood represented embers from the Saturday night fire, permitted the Sunday night fire to gain a decisive head start on the city fire department. The fire jumped the South Branch of the Chicago River before midnight. Dry winds rapidly drove it in a northeasterly direction. By 1:30 A.M. the central business district, including the courthouse, post office, and other buildings, was leveled. By 2:30 A.M. the fire had crossed the main part of the Chicago River and begun to consume the North Side section, including the waterworks, which were destroyed by 3:30 A.M. Once the waterworks were gone, the entire firefighting capacity of the city was eliminated. Desperate efforts to contain the fire, including attempts to make a breakfire by blowing up buildings before they caught fire, were unsuccessful. Unchecked, the fire burned across the North Side and to the east, recrossed the Chicago River along the waterfront, and completed the destruction of the South Side. Near midnight on Monday, October 9, the fire was burning itself out when rain accomplished what was beyond the reach of humans (Clevely 1958, Cromie 1958, Nash 1976).

The following first-person accounts are taken from Angle's *The Great Chicago Fire*, a compendium of letters and diaries from the Chicago Historical Society archives. They depict, as clearly as photographs, the forces involved in such a conflagration. Jonas Hutchinson, a lawyer and notary public, wrote to his mother that Monday:

This has been an eventful day. . . . What a sight: a sea of fire, the heavens all ablaze, the air filled with burning embers, the wind blowing fiercely & tossing fire brands in all directions, thousands upon thousands of people rushing frantically about, burned out of shelter, without food, the rich of yesterday poor today, destruction everywhere — is it not awful?

The fire moved over the city so quickly that even those aware of it did not at first perceive the danger to themselves or their households. George Howland, the principal of Central High School, wrote a friend in Massachusetts:

I noticed the fire soon after getting home from church Sunday evening, and supposing it a continuation of the one the night before, retired about 12 as calm as usual. . . . Hearing the remarks of some people in the street [I] concluded to go down. The sparks were falling like snowflakes, and the wind blowing a gale, but no more, I thought, than the previous night. I went over [to] the South Side and found it [the fire] then on the courthouse. People thought that as it had got among the brick & stone it would be retarded. I went back . . . when my brother, who had been driven out, came in and told me that I would have to move. I told him I thought not as it was past us already, and told him that I would make him a cup of coffee. . . . I was just pouring my coffee, when hearing a crackling, I went to the door and found the roof all on fire. . . . Engines seemed entirely useless. The long tongues of flame would dart out over a whole block, then come back & lap it all up clean. Iron & stone seemed to come down as in a blast furnace.

One final eyewitness account, that of Mrs. Aurelia King, wife of a wholesale clothing merchant, vividly describes the physical nature of the event:

At one o'clock we were awakened by shouts of people in the streets declaring the city was on fire — but then the fire was far away on the south side of the river. Mr. King went quite leisurely over town, but soon hurried back with the news that the court-house, Sherman House, Post Office, Tremont House, and all the rest of the business portion of the city was in flames, and thought he would go back and keep an eye on his store. He had scarcely been gone fifteen minutes when I saw him rushing back with news that everything was burning, that the bridges were on fire, and the North Side was in danger. From that moment the flames ran in our direction, coming faster than a man could run. The rapidity was almost incredible, the wind blew hurricane, the air was full of burning boards and shingles flying in every direction, and falling everywhere around us. It was all so sudden we did not realize our danger until we saw our Water Works (which were beyond us) were burning, when we gave up all hope, knowing that the water supply must soon be cut off. . . . It was 2 o'clock in the morning when I fled with my little children clinging to me, fled literally in a shower of fire.

In the end, the fire had leveled nearly every building in a 3⅓-square-mile area in the heart of the city, destroyed property valued at $200,000,000, left one-third of the city population homeless, and killed about 300 people. The burned buildings carried approximately $88,000,000 in insurance and eventually $45–50 million in claims was paid. Despite the extent of the destruction, business began to resume almost immediately. Tuesday morning, less than twelve hours after the fire had been extinguished, lumber arrived in Chicago, and rebuilding started.

The Great Chicago Fire, like the San Francisco earthquakes and resultant fires of 1907 and 1989, illustrates the tremendous effect fire can have on a major city, even one designed according to the fire codes of the day and prepared — insofar as possible — for disaster. We particularly remember such fires because of their effects on many lives and properties and their effects on our imaginations: if Chicago can go up in flames, then surely no city is entirely safe, including whichever one we inhabit. This force and random quality of fire, so vividly described by the Chicago survivors, are undoubtedly the basis for the easy popularity of fire as a cinematic device in contemporary popular film-making.

Burns in Aesthetics and Art

In real life, most real evil is committed by "normal" people, normal on the outside, at least. And some, like murderer Ted Bundy, are extraordinarily good looking. The responses that I (JAP) see in my plastic surgery patients who are facially scarred are more likely to be depression, shyness, and sorrow — mixed with hope that surgery will undo the damage, or provide enough change so they will not be stared at in public — not violent, melodramatic urges for violence and revenge. Evidently writers and moviemakers enjoy — and we encourage them by our support — explaining evil by giving it an external, specific, and unusual cause, such as a burn. How clear this makes good and evil! How clearly separate such victims must be from you and me!

In art, fire images have played an important role. Alice Turner's highly illustrated *History of Hell* amply documents the artistic vision of fire represented in European art history. The religious images expressed in those paintings and murals reflect the religious and intellectual preoccupations with time, sin, and punishment. Contemporary art, breaking away from religious sponsorship, usually reflects more secular values and themes. The pop icons of Andy Warhol and abstract works of Jackson Pollock avoid fire and flames. Sharon Romm (1986), a plastic surgeon, in her article "Art in Burns" describes a modern burn painting, "El Quemado" ("The Burning Man"). This 1955 oil by Mexican artist Rufino Tamayo presents a figure with upstretched arms and hands, flames swirling about and above him while he stares out of the canvas. Tamayo says he had "nothing special in mind" and has never experienced, seen, or known a burn survivor. Yet the painting accurately portrays the anguish of being burned. An artist may deny the connection but many others report being compelled by news photos of Hiroshima and Nagasaki or images from Europe (Dresden, for example) to portray such anguish. The powerful, skeletal, nearly radiant images collected in Marshall Arisman's *Heaven Departed* (1989) show an anguish much like the Tamayo painting. *Impact* (see Figure 18), for example, shows a silhouetted figure, arms outstretched, coming down a road, with an intense mushroom shaped light filling the background; it recalls the Ut photo from Vietnam.

Health care providers can repair seriously burned patients, but rarely restore them fully to their previous appearance and mental state. Instead all of us can imagine more creatively and empathetically the burdens burn survivors carry, both in body and in mind. Often these burdens are unspoken. It is difficult to put the burden into words. Patients often have not brought them fully to consciousness. And on another level we may not want to hear about what we intuit to be a dreadful experience. It is also very likely that we have not asked, and therefore not given them permission to speak of such things.

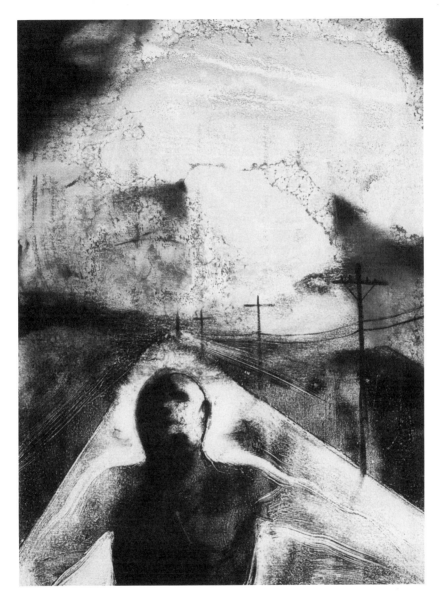

Figure 18. Marshall Arisman, *Impact*, from his collection of paintings and prints, *Heaven Departed*. Tokyo Designers School, 1989; used by permission of the artist.

The sorts of images discussed in this chapter may have influenced both patients' and healers' perceptions of fire, burns, and damaged selves. These images may have also influenced family and friends, who, in turn, influence patients. Since such a commercially successful symbol in the popular media is unlikely to change, we need to be aware of its pervasive influence and to work past it.

The approach of David Tepplica, for example, is instructive. A plastic surgeon, he has created an exhibit of photographs entitled "Scars of Childhood." In his introduction to the exhibit he writes, "Burn injury . . . remains one of the leading causes of childhood death and disfigurement in the United States. . . . [A]n estimated one million children are injured and 3,000 die each year as a result of burn trauma. For those who survive, permanent scarring, physical deformity, social isolation and emotional trauma linger well beyond the initial tragedy." The photographs, taken by Tepplica of his own burn patients, depict the burn center and difficult treatments his patients undergo — images rarely seen outside their dramatic context. We come to see caregivers not only as healers to their patients but also as empathetic witnesses to their patients' ordeals. The exhibition of these photos, not just at burn meetings, but in public spaces (the Empire State Building in New York, the U.S. Army Medical Department Museum in San Antonio, and others) highlights the humanity of the victims, makes real the risk of injury, and increases awareness of our responsibility for these individuals. To this end, the presentations have been cosponsored by the Phoenix Society for Burn Survivors and by firefighter groups; sometimes the presentations are accompanied by illustrated programs on burn prevention and fire safety.

Given the pervasive imagery of guilt and evil we have seen attached to burns, caregivers have an obligation to look at the possible readings patients may give to burns and to be especially alert to depression, self-blame, and infantile regressions. Caregivers should also examine whether they separate the patients from their own social spheres as different, somehow "lower," or "damaged goods," or just plain stupid. Such attitudes will negatively influence medical care. Clearly physical care alone — the healing of the flesh wound — is not enough. It is not enough only to catch Icarus in his fall; we must talk to him, learn of his inner turmoil, and help him find peace. Often it is artists — whether cinematic, literary, or graphic — who can present the horrors of being burned with a full emotional range. Some of these will be the easier clichés of popular culture, while others will be more carefully worked and deeply insightful. Society at large has the challenge of overcoming the negative images of burns and envisioning the person apart from the disfigurement of the burn scars.

Chapter Seven
Honey or Acid?
A Short History of Burn Care

The history of burn care is a micro-history of the care of wounds and of changing military surgical practices. The earliest battle wounds were largely caused by cutting traumas (spears, swords, arrows); burns were typically domestic or incidental. The invention of gunpowder opened a new era of mass casualties, and of wounds caused by blast and burn. The later addition of vehicles powered by petroleum products — tanks, planes, helicopters — added direct-flame burns to the list of common military casualties. Indeed the observations of intelligent practitioners in the laboratory of the battlefield and funding from the military establishment made possible progress in the care of such victims. Paré, Buck, Gilles, and MacIndoe are some of the great names associated with advances in burn, and hence wound, care. In this chapter we will review the history of burn treatments, emphasizing their wide range and underlying philosophical assumptions.

In his classic textbook *Principles of Surgery* (1872) Samuel Gross gives what is still a truism about burns:

There are few accidents which are of more common occurrence than burns and scalds, or which entail a greater amount of suffering and deformity. The progress of civilization, and the improvements in the arts and sciences, have greatly multiplied their frequency and severity, and call for corresponding attention on the part of the surgeon. . . . From what I have seen of these lesions, I am satisfied that few practitioners understand their character, or treat them with the success of which they are capable. One reason, perhaps, of this is that every one of them has a remedy for them, and that hardly any two agree as to the kind of treatment best adapted to their relief. (593)

Regrettably, this statement, more than a century old, still applies to some aspects of contemporary burn medical and surgical management. The availability of multiple remedies and the absence of standardized, universally accepted treatment regimens indicates not just a lack of consensus but a corresponding failure in developing a treatment which is clearly superior to any of the others currently available. Modern medical knowledge of burns and their sequelae has certainly improved since Gross's time, there is still no consensus about preferred strategies for treatment of systemic effects, local treatment of the burn wounds, and the timing and staging of surgery. The reasons for this variety are largely historical in the long term—the many strategies that have been proposed—and in the short term. Individual units and physicians have their own favored ways of treatment; sometimes they scornfully refer to treatments of other units as "N.I.H." ("Not Invented Here"). On the one hand, it may be regrettable that all units do not follow a "gold standard" of optimum treatment; on the other, since there is no agreement on what this standard would be, it may be good that a creative ferment is exploring a variety of approaches. Ultimately either "the best" will emerge or, more likely, a range of effective treatments from which physicians may choose, based on patient needs, personal preferences, and other factors. Fakhry et al. (1995) have shown that standards of care vary widely from burn unit to unit in the United States. Internationally, they vary even more widely from country to country, given economic status, religious beliefs, and access to materials.

The earliest written description of specific treatment for burns is found in the Ebers Papyrus, where a salve is prepared using "sntr," possibly the resin of the turpentine tree:

Sntr-resin, one part
Honey, one part
Anoint with it.

This salve was applied along with magical incantation. Based on what we know today, the incantation itself may have had a soothing effect, and the remedy itself may have even had a therapeutic benefit. This, in contrast to other later remedies, was at least not harmful. The incantation included a long general preamble used when any remedy was about to be applied, followed by a chant specific to the burn wound.
    One such chant is:

Your son, Horus has burned himself in the desert.
Is water here?
There is no water here.
Water is in my mouth
A Nile is between my thighs,
I have come to put out the fire.
Flow out, burn. (Majno, 128)

This chant acknowledges the intense thirst characteristic of a major burn injury, caused by fluid shifts. Not only does water stop the burning process when applied as a coolant directly onto the burn wound, but fluid replacement helps to prevent burn shock. Not until the twentieth century have burn doctors investigated and applied this important principle. The treatment of burns now must include the quick replacement of enough water, either by mouth or by intravenous line, to produce a "Nile between the thighs," or a high urine flow.

Resins and tree sap, including myrrh, are among the oldest remedies known; they occur regularly as topical ingredients around the world even now, especially in areas where cost and lack of access prevent the use of contemporary remedies. A biblical reference to sap (balm in Gilead) as a remedy is

I am wounded at the sight of my people's wound,
I go like a mourner, overcome with horror.
Is there no balm in Gilead, no physician there?

Go up into Gilead and fetch balm,
O virgin people of Egypt.
You have tried many remedies, all in vain:
No skin shall grow over your wounds. (Jeremiah 8: 22; 46: 11)

The implication is that, without the balm, no healing will occur.

Herodotus (480 B.C.E.) describes how the Persians used myrrh to treat wounds. The Hippocratic books mention use of myrrh 54 times, making it the most commonly employed resin. Celsus, in the first century C.E., describes a lotion of myrrh and wine for the treatment of burns. Pliny the Elder in *Natural History* (77 C.E.) describes a variety of recipes containing plant extracts, wine, and other mineral, animal, and vegetable material collected from Greek and Latin sources (Scarborough 1983). Guido Majno has evaluated some of these treatments, finding that many were not harmful and some may even have had salutary effects (Majno 1975). We know today that substances like honey, myrrh, copper sulfate, and wine have antibacterial properties and are not toxic in low concentrations.

In early times, however, there was no concept of anti-infective activity, nor understanding of the natural process of wound healing. Substances were designated because of the traditional magical authority of priests, healers, or revered texts, not so much because of observed empirical efficacy. In general, the importance of observation emphasized in the Hippocratic teachings and the cause-and-effect philosophy of Aristotle did not become the official method to determine treatments until centuries later. Indeed a rigid adherence to formulae and excessive reverence for established texts impeded medical progress. Galen's encyclopedic writings on the practice of medicine, for example, went unchallenged for nearly 1,000 years, although folk medicines of many sorts evolved by trial and error.

In 1491 Johannes DeKetham was recommending olive oil, honeycomb, Arabic gum, and incense, all ingredients recommended in the earliest Egyptian writings. These substances were probably harmless at worst and possibly therapeutic at best — at least according to our contemporary understanding of wound healing. Oils such as olive oil, grease, and the wax of honeycomb would prevent bandages from sticking, and they do not spoil readily. Honey, wine, myrrh, copper sulfate, and vinegar all have antibacterial properties that are still valued and used today. Lint and other fabrics would absorb drainage from the wound, including pus when the wound inevitably became infected. Indeed what distinguished the approach to wound healing until the end of the nineteenth century was an expectation of infection. The presence of pus, or suppuration, was so regular a feature of healing that it was believed to be necessary to the completion of the healing process. Redness and swelling with heat and pain (first described by Hippocrates) followed all wounds, as noted by Celsus (*De Medicina*) in 25 C.E. (cited in Scarborough, Harkins, Majno, Caldwell).

Various writers distinguished between pus that was beneficial and pus that indicated a fatal infection. The first — so-called "laudable pus" — was the thick creamy whitish pus that we know today characterizes staphylococcal infections. These organisms, normal colonizers of the skin, when localized to the wound may be safely treated with only local wound care. The healthy person will have sufficient immune competence to fight the infection with normal body defense mechanisms. Watery, foul-smelling, brownish or greenish pus, a result of infections with streptococcal bacteria — or what are known as the gram negative organisms (such as *E. coli*, *Pseudomonas* organisms, or clostridial bacteria) — are capable of overcoming host resistance; even with the use of topical and systemic antibiotics, these can be fatal. Before sepsis was understood and treated with modern approaches, such infections would have been nearly universally fatal.

Although Hypocrites, Galen, and early practitioners of surgery described wounds and their management in some detail, even using the mechanism of injury and its effects on the flesh to predict outcomes, they did not discuss burns as a separate category of wound. Rather, they understood burns as a treatment modality: a burn applied to a wound might stop hemorrhage. This use of burning to treat wounds, largely an ironic concept to us, continued in various forms into the twentieth century. Techniques used by American Indians included the application of hot stones, glowing needles, or hot shells. Tibetan monks poured a mixture of sulfur and saltpeter into wounds and set fire to it.

The introduction of gunpowder in the thirteenth century changed the nature of war wounds and significantly increased injury-related deaths. Giovanni de Vigo, in the sixteenth century, was so struck by this that he postulated the presence of a toxin in gunpowder burns. In the eighteenth century, gunpowder was actually placed in amputation stumps and ignited, although the older method, direct burning with a torch, was used more often.

The revolutionary idea that burning might be bad for a wound was first put forth by Ambroise Paré, a French military surgeon of the sixteenth century. His education had been at the Hôtel Dieu in Paris, where the works of de Vigo were studied. De Vigo theorized that gun powder made shot wounds poisonous and recommended pouring seething (i.e., heated) elder-oil and theriaca (an antidote) into the wound (Cockshott 1956). During his first tour as a military surgeon, Paré accompanied the French troops into northern Italy and saw many wounds. After that war, he wrote vividly of his experiences in his first publication:

To avoid doing anything crazy, and knowing that this treatment would be very painful to the victims, I decided to wait until I had seen what the other surgeons did. They actually made the oil as hot as possible and dabbed it on the wound. I then took heart and did the same. But my oil ran out and I had to apply a healing salve made of egg-white, rose-oil, and turpentine.

The next night I slept badly, plagued by the thought that I would find the men dead whose wounds I had failed to burn, so I got up early to visit them. To my great surprise those treated with salve felt little pain, showed no inflammation or swelling, and had passed the night rather calmly—while the ones on which seething oil had been used lay in high fever with aches, swelling and inflammation around the wound. At this, I resolved never again to cruelly burn poor people who had suffered shot wounds. (Haeger 1988, 105)

His opposition to burning extended to the cautery iron, then the method used to stop bleeding from the stumps of amputations. Paré's alternative was the direct ligation of the vessels at the time of surgery. This radical departure was not accepted by subsequent authoritative surgeons, however, for several centuries. For instance, Fabricius Hildanus (1560–1634) recommended the use of a red hot knife to sear the vessels during amputation (Shedd 1958). Richard Wisemen (circa 1676) described Paré's method but still recommended the use of a "royal styptic" or actual cautery. Stump burning was not abandoned until the nineteenth century, when various methods of ligature became widely accepted.

Another contribution by Paré to the understanding of burn injuries was his observation that the pain of a burn was related to its depth. He wrote, "A deep burn having caused hard scabs is not so painful as a superficial one, as is proved by daily experience in respect of those who are cauterized. For just after cauterization, they only feel a little pain. For a great combustion removes the feeling" (Harkins 1942, 107). A third major contribution made by Paré to modern burn care was his comparisons of different treatments and their outcomes—the forerunner of modern clinical trials. Sigerist—in a charming Renaissance translation—relates Paré's discovery of the efficacy of onions in the treatment of burns:

One of the Marshall of *Montejan* his Kitchin boyes fell by chance into a Caldron of oyle being even almost boyling hot; I being called to dresse him, went to the next Apothecaries to fetch refrigerating medicines commonly used in this case: there was present by chance a certaine old countrey woman, who hearing that I desired medicines for a burne, perswaded mee at the first dressing, that I should lay to raw Onions beaten with a little salt: for so I should hinder the breaking out of blisters or pustules, as shee had found by certaine and frequent experience. Wherefore I thout good to try the force of her Medicine upon this greasy scullion. I the next day found those places of his body where to the Onions lay to be free from blisters but the other parts which they had not touched, to be all blistered. (Sigerist 1944, 144)

This observation led Paré to test the onion remedy again, applying it in the case of a guard with gunpowder burns of the hands and face, "I being called, laid the Onions beaten as I formerly told you, to one half of his face, and to the other half I laid medicines usually applyed to burnes. At the second dressing I observed the part dressed with the Onions quite free from blisters and excoriation, the other being troubled with both: whereby I gave credit to the Medicine." Paré continued his experiments with onions, comparing the one remedy against others until he was thoroughly convinced that the method was superior to other recommendations. Paré was widely translated and his ideas accepted. As with many folk remedies, the efficacy of onions is being confirmed through an analysis of the active ingredients. Dorsch (1990) and his colleagues have identified seven different synthetic thiosulfinates in onion extract that inhibit the action of human granulocytes. These anti-inflammatory agents reduce the activity and presence of white cells (pus) in wounds. Their work (1989) has also demonstrated that onion extract has an anti-histamine action that may reduce platelet action and have efficacy in asthma.

One of the earliest English works on burns was a monograph by the surgeon William Clowes, *A Profitable and Necessarie Booke of Observations for all Those that are Burnt with the Flame of Gunpowder* (1637). Although his remedies were largely derived from Paré (including the use of onions and salt) or earlier European writers, his case histories are colorful and detailed and reveal that more injuries derived from careless handling of gunpowder than from actual gunshot wounds (Shedd 1958). The introduction of gunpowder in warfare changed the nature of the injuries sustained in battle: all subsequent military medical texts include burns as an important subject.

In Italy, Gaspare Tagliacozzi, Professor of Anatomy at Bologna, published his historic work *De Curatorum Chirurgia* (1597), in which he describes numerous innovative reconstructive techniques, including the use of skin grafts for burns and other injuries. In England, Fabricius Hildanus published *De Combustionibus* (1607), a treatise on burns. A popular text, it was republished through several editions during the next 75 years. Hildanus was the first to classify burns into three degrees, "levissimam, mediocrem et insignam." The book describes numerous remedies for burns (again including onions and salt), as well as treatments such as splints and pulleys designed to reverse burn scar contractures. The illustrations showing burn scar contractures of the hand are detailed but incorrect, demonstrating radial deviations of finger contractures when ulnar deviations are the usual result; that is, the fingers are pulled toward the sides of the hand away from the thumb (Robotti 1990). Richard Wiseman, the best-known English surgeon of his time, was considered the first to separate the practice of surgery from the barber-surgeon school. In 1676 he published *Several Chirurgicall Treatises.* He observed "If the burn be superficial it raiseth the cuticle up in blisters: if it goes deeper into the skin, it causes an exchar: if it burns deeper into the flesh, the force of fire makes a hard crust with contraction." He also observed that a superficial burn is painful while a deeper burn is not. His observations were accurate, and some were based on personal experience: while dressing a gangrenous limb with turpentine (the standard remedy of the day) he accidentally ignited the dressing and burned his own hand (Harkins 1942).

In 1792 David Cleghorn, an Edinburgh brewer, published a work entitled *Medical Facts and Observations.* His practical treatment of burns came from personal experience in treating workers injured in his breweries. He observed that purgation by repeated enemas—a common practice—was harmful to the burn patient, a view repeated by Hornby in 1833 (Cockshott 1956). Although Cleghorn's work was admired and he was considered the expert on burns of his time, this admonition did not halt the practice of purgation, which surely further weakened patients. The practice of "heroic" medicine continued into the nineteenth century with treatments such as bleeding with leeches or cuts and purging either by inducing emesis or by enemas, despite the observations of Cleghorn.

In his *Essay on Burns* (1797), Edward Kentish commented on the numerous prescriptions for burns contained in Fabricius's work. This English physician noticed that some cures were worse than the wound: "I presume one of the great causes of error is the assigning to various applications the cure of slight burns, some of which no doubt would have got well without any, and perhaps much sooner than with those which were used." Kentish recommended the use of oil of turpentine for burn treatment, based on the observation that a burn looks much like gangrene. His most original contribution to burn care, however, was in the use of pressure dressings, which he claimed reduced pain and blisters. Furthermore, his text was the first to concern itself not with war-related injuries but with the care of civilians, in this case Scottish coal miners. The dedication in the frontispiece of his book remains pertinent:

I am afraid the following remark will be found true as it is extraordinary, that during a period exceeding 600 years that the coal trade has flourished in this neighborhood not a single remark upon the subject has preserved upon the record, though during that period some of the first surgical and medical men in the kingdom have had the phenomena constantly before their eyes. What causes can be assigned to such inattention to the interests of humanity? Ignorance and prejudice on the part of people, and disgust on that of the faculty; these appear to be the principal causes why so little attention has been paid on the part of the practitioners. (Shedd 1958, 1030)

The ability of observers like Paré, Cleghorn, and Kentish to distinguish between the recommended efficacy of treatments and their observed effects represents the true beginning of scientific inquiry in the management of burns. It also signals the changing relationship between practitioners of medicine and works considered to be the canon of medicine—Celsius, Galen, and others—whose doctrine could now be challenged and revised.

Thomas Parkinson in 1799 reported on the use of alcohol in the treatment of burns. What distinguished his report from those of many others prescribing remedies is his attempt to provide a rational basis and mechanism of action for the efficacy of alcohol. He begins by discussing why he is dissatisfied with other recommended treatments, then says of his method:

as it has not only novelty, but facts, to recommend it. . . . I am disposed to attribute the good effects, which the application of spirit of wine produces, principally to the degree of cold generated by evaporation; and, possibly, this may be still further improved by employing vitriolic ether instead of spirit of wine. . . . I find this very generally of sufficient efficacy to prevent, or to destroy inflammation; frequently to preserve much skin which has been injured; and, ultimately, to render little more than a mild cerate of wax and oil necessary to accomplish the cure. (Harkins, 9)

As burns became a specific area of inquiry, literature began to appear that distinguished mechanism and severity of injury, and examined treatments in an increasingly systematic manner. Guillaume Dupuytren, an astute French surgeon who is best known today for his description of palmar fibrosis (Dupuytren's contracture), provided the first truly scholarly approach to burns (Robotti, 177, Harkins, 10). He reviewed the history of burn care and surgery and rediscovered the work of Tagliacozzi; he then referred to the grafting for burns as the "Italian" method. Dupuytren provided the first detailed method of classifying burns into six degrees, based on the depth of structures involved from skin down to bone. In addition to recognizing the relationship of depth of burn injury to its seriousness and possible outcomes, Dupuytren also described the natural history of burn illness, dividing the course into four stages: "the life of the patient may be endangered successively at four different periods, the period of irritation, period of inflammation, period of suppuration and period of exhaustion" (Hawkins, 20). These distinctions remain valid today in that they correspond to what are now recognized as distinct physiologic responses to the initial severe injury: the fluid shifts that follow initial survival, the inevitable infections that develop after five to ten days, and the final results of hypermetabolism, when patients lose weight unless their enormous caloric requirements are met. Death can occur at any of these stages; later advances in burn care and enhanced survival became possible only when the unique character of each stage was recognized and properly managed.

In its turn, America also produced textbooks including recommendations for the treatment of burns. John Jones, the first Professor of Surgery at

Kings College (now Columbia University) published *Plain Concise Practical Remarks on the Treatment of Wounds and Fractures* in 1775, in time to make it the standard text for the Revolutionary Army. His description of burns by degrees corresponds to modern terminology, and he used his classification to suggest different treatments. The least burns, first degree, were treated with the spirit of wine. Burns that produce blisters, second degree, were treated with linseed oil or a wax of oil (cerate). Because deeper burns harm "the true skin, and membrane adipose down to the muscles affected, and slough away, a different mechanism of treatment is to be made use of" (John Jones, quoted in Stark 1975, 510). The burned tissue was allowed to slough away, leaving an open, granulating surface. This surface was then covered with an ointment consisting of hog's lard, boiled thorn-apple leaves, and wax, in a consistency that would adhere to the wound, protect it from pain, and not melt away on warm days. Jones characterized this period of healing as the state of inflammation and described the slow start of cicatrization (the process of healing by contraction and epithelialization) as "long enough to tire both the patient and surgeon, for, where the burn or scald is very extensive, the elongation of the sound skin is produced with great difficulty, and is extremely apt to break down upon the slightest occasion" (Stark, 510). Again, these words are still accurate.

In Edinburgh, in 1833, Sir George Ballingall published *Outlines of Military Surgery*, in which he described the natural history of a burn patient vividly and accurately: "he stinks from causes which we cannot explain . . . sinking in hectic state, exhausted by a profuse discharge of matter from an extensive suppurating surface." He maintained the traditional recommendations of purging and blood letting but offered no specific cure for his observed afflictions (Shedd 1958, 1099).

Just as war provided astute observers such as Paré with tests of their theories and methods of treating large numbers of casualties, the industrial revolution created similar opportunities for those (such as Cleghorn and Kentish) treating occupational injuries. One example is Dr. John Roebuck, the owner of Carron Iron Foundries in Scotland, who developed a remedy which was a mixture of linseed oil and lime water. This "carron oil" became the standard formula in use from the 1700s through the end of the nineteenth century (Moncrief 1971). Another example is G. Passavant, who, in 1857, treated 13 survivors of an explosion at a pyrotechnic laboratory at Frankfort am Main by using saline baths—a treatment also recommended by Dupuytren (Robotti, 177). The reported success of such treatments by Roebuck and Passavant and their ensuing popularization were possible because publication was increasingly recognized as important, worthwhile, and authoritative: other practitioners who read about these treatments and techniques began to use them. Thus carron oil and saline treatment entered common practice within years, changing canons of practice that had existed for centuries. The willingness to accept change and the increasing desire to treat based on evidence of success rather than doctrine provided the intellectual climate necessary for the great changes that occurred in medical thinking and practice later in the nineteenth century.

The nineteenth century was an era of almost explosive progress in medicine. In its opening years, hospitals were death houses where pain and infection were guaranteed to accompany injury and surgery, and medicine in general could claim little efficacy from its treatments. Bleeding and purging were still commonly practiced as therapies, and people practiced medicine without formal education or regulation. Academic medicine made progress in accurate recognition of disease and illness and gained significant insight into human anatomy and physiology, but it contributed little to effective treatments, let alone actual cures. The nineteenth century—with its discoveries of general anesthesia by Morton and others and of microorganisms and their role in disease and fermentation by Koch and Pasteur, and the practice of antisepsis by Semmelweiss and Lister—provided the foundation upon which burn care could become humane and effective.

What is perhaps even more remarkable is that surgery flourished before these discoveries, that practitioners and patients had the courage to proceed. M. C. Furnell, in publishing his observations on the first use of chloroform anesthesia in England, recalls the first operation he witnessed, one without anesthesia. He describes the patient as repulsive, a result of a childhood burn injury that resulted in contractures. These caused her head to be drawn down onto her chest, with her lips pulled down so that she drooled constantly (see Figure 19). She consented to an operation to release the scar tissue and transplant skin from her arm into the cicatrix (scar). He then describes the procedure:

The patient was tied to the operating table, as was customary in those days but before many minutes of the operation had elapsed her cries and entreaties to be untied and allowed to remain as she was were the most frightful that can be imagined. As the operation, which was necessarily a lengthy and slow one, proceeded, her cries became more terrible, first one and then another student fainted, and ultimately all but a determined few had left the theater, unable to stand the distressing scene. (Furnell 1877)

The rapidity with which anesthesia was introduced reflects the speed of communication possible in the mid-nineteenth century. Morton first used ether in Boston in October 1846. In December Robert Liston used it in London for amputating a leg, and in January 1847, Heyfelder used it in Germany. By the end of 1847 chloroform was being used by James Simpson for obstetrics in Edinburgh. Thus in less than a year a new technique with modifications had been tested on both continents, even revised and adapted to new applications and with new drugs (Pernick 1988).

The acceptance and introduction into common practice that charac-

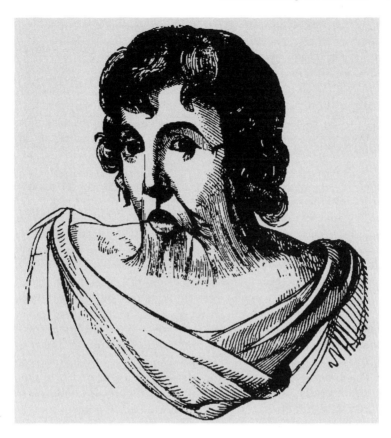

Figure 19. Cicatrices of the face and neck. This lithograph, originally from Gordun Buck, has been reprinted in many places. Scars like this, similar to that seen on the foot in Figure 6, were not uncommon in the pre-modern era and may still be seen in many parts of the world; they can pull the chin down to the chest, evert the lower eyelids, and hold the mouth permanently open. Samuel Gross, *A System of Surgery*, vol. 1 (Philadelphia: Henry Lee, 1872), 595.

terized anesthesia is in striking contrast to the strong resistance exhibited, especially in the U.S., to the ideas of Joseph Lister. Aseptic technique, based on a belief in the germ theory, was not widely accepted or practiced for more than thirty years after Lister's first published reports appeared. In the nineteenth century American medicine was an unorganized cluster of competing schools: allopathic, hydropathic, homeopathic, chiropractic, and even anti-professional movements like the Thompsonians, who preached "every man his own doctor," as well as religious healing movements like

Christian Science. Hundreds of small, uncredentialed schools graduated "doctors" who had no practical medical experience or scientific education, and did not need a license to practice medicine.

Eventually, the allopathic approach — which incorporated European educational principles, the study of Greek, Latin, and the humanities, with anatomy, physiology, and clinical training in medicine, surgery, obstetrics, and so forth — began to "professionalize" health care. This model of medicine emerged as the dominant medical model by the end of the nineteenth century and was validated by the Flexner Report of 1910. State licensure, accreditation of medical schools, the establishment of professional societies, and the advent of effective therapies combined to transform American medicine into the sophisticated, scientific practice we know today.

The development of professional medicine affected all aspects of medical practice, burn care no less than other specialties. By the end of the century, skin grafting was being performed, and burns were treated as physiological injuries, not just as wounds. Burn shock was recognized as the chief cause of early burn death, but treatment was still confined largely to the burned skin on the assumption that proper care of the wound would reduce burn shock. Moyer, in 1953, reviewed eight articles reporting mortality rates in series of large burns, showing that the survival of patients was steadily increasing with improved techniques. Sneve, for example, advocated the administration of large volumes of 0.9 percent sodium chloride (NaCl) by vein or mouth in 1905. This treatment represents the first authenticated report in the literature of survival of a deep burn of more than 25 percent total body surface area (TBSA). Weidenfield, in Vienna, reported a 100 percent mortality for 41 burns treated by the exposure method (open dry wound) in 1902, but modification of his method (occlusive dressing and small amounts of 0.9 percent NaCl up to three liters), reduced this mortality to 90 percent. Using acetate powder and large volumes of saline solution, Sneve reported 13 survivors of a total 24 treated, a 54 percent mortality. Further reports indicated similar survival rates through 1950.

Survival of patients with these larger burns required that the wounds be treated surgically: Leaving large injuries to heal spontaneously by granulation, contracture, and reepithelialization not only prolonged patient recovery, but also resulted in disfiguring scars and extensive deformity. Skin grafting, first reported by the ancient Hindus, rediscovered and performed by Tagliacozzi, and reported in the German literature in 1823, was necessary for larger injuries. Although Warren Mason, a prominent Boston surgeon, reported in 1843 a graft taken from the thigh to the nose, grafting was not popularized until Reverdin's breakthrough while working in 1872 as a house officer in the Hospital Necker under the direction of the great French physiologist Félix Jacques Guyon. Reverdin described using tiny pieces of epithelium for grafting, a technique that became the more widely practiced, perhaps because of a higher success rate of these "pinch grafts." The use of larger and thicker pieces of skin for grafting were reported by Ollier, Thiersch, Wolfe, and Krause, but general use of these grafts was limited by the technical difficulty of harvesting them. Vilray Blair, James Barrett Brown, and John Staige Davis used skin grafts to close burns and other large wounds, but their success depended largely on their personal skill at using large sharpened knives to slice thin sheets of skin, including some dermis with the epidermis (Padgett 1942). The pinch graft — using a small hook to lift up skin while slicing it off — was a simple freehand approach that did not rely on the skill of the operator. Not until Padgett invented the dermatome in 1939 did the use of large, thin pieces of skin for grafting become widely practiced (see Figure 20).

During World War I, with the use of tanks, airplanes, and motor vehicles to move troops and supplies, burns caused by exploding fuel tanks became a major medical concern. In England a specialized burn treatment facility was opened to provide concentrated care of the burn injuries sustained by airmen. Although the first specialized burn unit had opened in England in 1854 (Wallace 1987), it was short-lived, being taken over for the care of other surgery patients almost immediately. This time the burn unit provided sustained care of the injured, with special attention to burns of the hands and face, areas typically not protected by the clothing worn by pilots and combatants. Archibald MacIndoe, the director of the unit, became one of the leading plastic and reconstructive surgeons of his time. Care of these patients took months, even years, but provided major advances in reconstructive techniques. The burn care advocated in the military manuals of the time did not, however, recommend the use of intravenous fluid unless there were associated wounds causing bleeding. The standard of care was that the patient should be kept warm and given morphine to reduce pain, and that the burn wounds be covered.

A typical goal of wound care during the first half of the twentieth century was to promote the formation of an occlusive crust over the wound to reduce fluid loss and mitigate infection. Occlusive dressing with paraffin, continued use of dressings with Carron oil (now defined as linseed oil and lemon soaked cotton), open-wound treatment with powders of acetate, or simply leaving wounds open to dry — these were the dominant forms of wound care. In Europe, advocates of continuous saline baths to the wounds reported good results, presumably by removing toxins from the burn wound and decreasing fluid lost across the burn site, but these did not gain adherents in the United States. Advocates of the dry-wound technique postulated that the firm, hard eschar (dead tissue) that formed over the wound acted as a replacement skin until healing or grafting could take place. In a logical extension of this theory, Edward Davidson (1925) reintroduced the use of tannic acid to burn care. Tannic acid was a component of many early burn treatments and remains a popular folk remedy today. In a comprehensive review of contemporary burn wound research, Davidson concluded

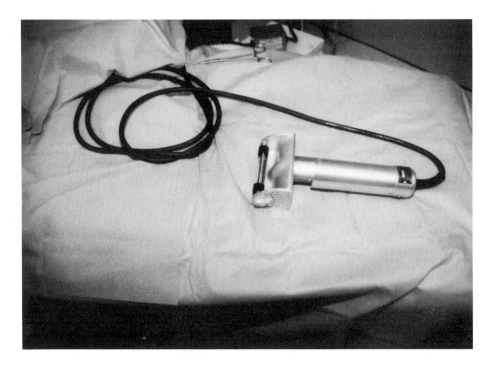

Figure 20. Electric dermatome. This dermatome, similar to a carpenter's plane, is used to debride and harvest skin. It can be adjusted to any thickness needed. Easier to use than the original Padgett drum dermatome, it and others like it enable any surgeon to harvest and use skin grafts. Photo by Jane Arbuckle Petro.

that tanning the wound reduces the toxemia of burn injury by stabilizing dangerous proteins in the burned skin. He wrote that the tanned tissue, referred to as "precipitated proteins," served to "provide a protective coating against chemical, bacterial, and mechanical action as well as against sensory and inflammatory irritation." He compared this action to that obtained by the picric acid previously used as a wound desiccant and pain reliever but which was accompanied by excessive toxicity, a property he had not observed with the use of tannic acid.

Davidson noted that earlier authors had advocated the earliest possible removal of burned skin, following which they recommended washing the wound with — of all things — gasoline; he concluded that such procedures were certain to hasten the death of already unstable burn patients. Delaying the excision and stabilizing the burn wound with tannic acid, he felt, would permit the patient's physiological recovery. The still-needed surgery would come later. Though authors before Davidson had proposed similar techniques, only Davidson — besides providing a comprehensive review of the burn literature up to that date — presented both animal data (his own and others') and detailed clinical case reports of burns in 17 patients treated by his method. This scholarly and rational paper is considered, with that of Frank Underhill (see below), to represent the best work of that era. American surgery, instead of imitating Europe, had matured enough to become a leader in the thought and practice of surgery in general and of burn care in particular.

The pioneering studies of Frank Underhill (1930) demonstrated that fluid loss caused by the burn injury rather than burn toxins was the cause of burn shock. In a healthy person blood pressure is maintained by multiple means; even in a sick or traumatized person, the intravascular space is flexible, taking on or returning blood to the vascular system in response to injury and illness. Thus blood pressure can remain steady over a wide range of volume gains or losses: up to 20 percent suddenly or 25 percent more slowly. This flexibility enables the body to protect critical organs — the brain, kidneys, and intestines — while delivering oxygen and energy sources. Burn shock results from the sudden fluid shift from the intravascular space leaking across the burn wound and into the extravascular spaces of the body elsewhere, especially the intestines, lungs, and soft tissues, even though they are not directly involved in the burn itself. The thirst that accompanies burns in a response by the central nervous system to this fluid shift.

Although burn shock and thirst were commonly known to accompany burn injury, it was not until Underhill described the fluid shift in acute burns that efforts to treat them included *calculated* fluid replacement. Underhill made his observations while caring for 20 survivors of the New Haven Rialto Theater fire in 1921. His paper, published in the *Journal of the American Medical Association* in 1930, is still quoted in the modern burn literature. His work exemplifies the modern tradition of the scientist/clinician: he included clinical observations of his patients, measuring their blood concentration and chemistries during the course of their recovery; he also offered observations from animal experiments which showed that the volume of fluid lost following a burn was proportionate to the surface area affected, and that up to 70 percent of the circulating blood volume might be lost during the first 24 hours after burn injury. While Sneve (1905) had advocated fluid replacement in burn patients of up to three liters of saline fluid, and others had noted a beneficial effect of transfusion or plasma replacement in burns, Underhill showed that four to eight liters might be required to replace what was actually a rapid emptying of the intravascular space in response to the burn, not just to circulating toxins.

Better attention to fluid balance, clean and sterile technique in wound care, and (later) the use of antibiotics to aid in the control of infection permitted longer survival of patients. Tannic acid probably was a superior wound care agent, certainly when compared with some previously recommended agents, such as turpentine, gasoline, mercury, white lead paint, or arsenical compounds; its use continued into World War II as a simple relatively safe method of wound care, especially if the patient could not be transported promptly. Later authors, however, noted significant toxicity to the liver associated with tannic acid; its use was abandoned in 1942, when it was confirmed to be the agent responsible for liver necrosis seen in some burns (Moncrief 1971).

In the era preceding World War II, burn care had made major advances. Shock was treated with fluids. Wound care was significantly improved, based on actual study of injuries and their relation to the patient. Such wound care included efforts to prevent infection, speed healing, and complete the healing process by skin grafting. Survival in cases of burns involving more than ¼ to ⅓ TBSA approached 50 percent and fatalities in cases of smaller burns became rare. These advances were to be important for military medicine; the number of burn casualties in World War I was reported to be 1 in 10 injuries, but for World War II, the proportion changed to 1 in 4, largely attributable to the wider use of petrochemicals. There were also larger numbers of civilian casualties, including burn victims, often from widespread non-military target bombing. Military funding for burn research led directly to the era of modern burn care, which includes a comprehensive medical approach to patient care in a dedicated unit specializing in burn management, reconstruction, and rehabilitation.

The first civilian population to benefit directly from increased military attention to burn injury was the city of Boston, site of the well-known Cocoanut Grove Fire in 1942. Previous civic experiences with fire in public places—such as the Iroquois Theater Fire in Chicago in 1903, where over 600 people, primarily women and children, died—did not result in permanent lessons in fire safety. Unmarked exits, locked emergency exits, flammable decorations, and poor crowd control, all recognized as significant factors in the 1903 catastrophe, contributed to the terrible fire disaster in Boston. In contrast to previous fire disasters where the event and the victims were largely forgotten, the experience of Boston and its survivors have earned a unique place in fire history. A combination of events—World War II, the presence in Boston of superb, competing medical institutions, and a recent civilian and military disaster drill—all provided an experiment in the management of burn injuries that was well staffed, thoroughly detailed, indeed wonderfully successful, although of course unplanned. The information gathered by the trained medical researchers and practitioners at Massachusetts General Hospital and Boston City Hospital permanently transformed the modern approach to burn care. In addition to new insights into smoke inhalation, fluid resuscitation, wound care and skin grafting, the experience allowed the chaplains and psychologists who cared for the surviving injured and the survivors of the deceased to recognize and treat posttraumatic stress disorder. After the war, this training was invaluable in the care of civilians who had survived concentration camps and soldiers who were prisoners of war. Furthermore, this new understanding led to today's acknowledgment that paramedics and other medical personnel are traumatized by mass casualty events and disasters, and that all such workers need debriefing to deal with the stress. A recent example is the bombing of the Alfred P. Murrah Federal Building in Oklahoma City; fire-fighters, rescuers, and medical personnel were all subjected to great stress, and trained psychologists and psychiatrists conducted critical incident debriefing for them.

Modern burn care owes much to the Cocoanut Grove fire disaster. The two hospitals receiving the patients, Massachusetts General Hospital and Boston City Hospital, had on their staffs individuals with sufficient experience treating burns that they knew which questions to ask, and, as a result of wartime, funded research projects that permitted them to test and validate their theories on the large influx of patients. At Boston City, Drs. Lund and Browder, attempting to quantify burn severity, developed their still used classification of burns based on the total body surface area, a classification that allows for triage and treatment decisions (see Figure 2). At Massachusetts General Hospital, Drs. Moore, Cope, and Levinson recognized the impact inhalation injury had on resuscitation and fluid requirements and studied the effect and effectiveness of new antibiotics on burn wound infection and healing (see Chapter 8). These clinical researchers, and the students who worked with them for the next three decades, became the modern scientists and burn care givers who have made possible the survival of "impossibly" injured people.

Part III
Modern Burn Care
Challenges to Patients, Families, and Caregivers

Chapter Eight
Contemporary Burn Care
*"They Have All These Neat Things
They Can Do Now"*

The technology contemporary western medical care can offer burn patients now includes an enormous range: transplantation, resuscitation, advanced life support, medications of enormous benefit (and toxicity), even diagnostic imaging tools such as PET scanning, which can show cognitive activity. All these — and many more — contribute to modern burn care, but, regrettably, do not always enhance it: U.S. care, for all of its high-tech orientation, has no better mortality levels than some low-tech care elsewhere in the world. Despite centralization of care in the United States through a network of burn *centers* (carrying out research, teaching, and patient care), burn *units* (providing teaching and care), and burn *beds* (burn care facilities), the overall mortality of burn victims is generally calculated at less than 5 percent of all burn injuries—about the same as that in China and Brazil. This similarity is especially dramatic when we consider the enormous differences in expenditures per patient. China, for example, reports survivals of burns in excess of 90 percent TBSA at a cost of less than $20,000 per patient (Jie 1992), while U.S. expenditures for similar survivals cost over $100,000. In Brazil, where the daily reimbursement in a burn center is $20 or less per day (compared to the U.S. cost of $1,000 per day) results are, once again, similar to our own (personal experience, JAP). An examination of these comparisons provides insight into such areas as the innate human capacities for survival, the differences in cultural and economic circumstances, and the differences of philosophy between high-tech medicine in the United States and high-practicality medicine in Brazil and China (see also Benmeir 1991 and Reig 1994).

The challenge of modern burn care is two-fold: (1) biological survival of the patient and (2) restoration of the behavioral and functional capacities following hospital discharge. The first aim includes treatment of ever larger and more complex burns (for example, the radiation burns of firefighters in the Chernobyl nuclear generator disaster) as well as all manner of high-energy trauma: plane, train, and car crashes with multiple injuries, burn, fractures, and ruptured viscera. The second challenge, at least in the theoretical ideal, is the full restoration of patients' functional capacity — in short, their ability to resume their pre-burn lives. Whether we can reach this goal is one of the major concerns of burn professionals, but the primary expenditure of resources puts the emphasis disproportionately on the first goal, including the acute phases of burn care, the glamorous and dramatic components of resuscitation, wound management, and infection control. Regrettably, less funding and research supports the development of rehabilitation and prevention.

In this chapter we will examine technologic advances in these two areas (survival and rehabilitation) since the end of World War II. We choose World War II as a turning point because of the impact wartime research had on burn care; not only the increased number of physicians and nurses trained in the surgical specialties but also the extended knowledge of war wounds, especially traumatic burns. As indicated earlier, U.S. Department of Defense research funding for burn care directly affected medical practice at the time of the Cocoanut Grove fire in 1942. Centralization of military burn care at the Brooke Army Hospitals Institute for Surgical Research (San Antonio, Texas) was a direct precursor of the modern U.S. system of civilian burn centers, many of whose leaders came from the young surgeons trained at Brooke during the wars that followed World War II.

The Patient and the Burn Center: The Case of Tim

Burn care can be illustrated in a number of ways. We could break down several individual cases and report their progress, report the newest advances in burn care as a continuation of the historical approach used in the preceding chapter, or select one outstanding case and follow it through, using the details of the singular as a stepping off point for the general. The advantages of the singular approach include narrative progress, human interest, detailed reflection. During the course of any given year in a burn center there are always a few cases that stand out, either for their horror (severity of the burn, deaths associated with the fire), the nature and personality of the patient or their family, or the nature of the accident causing the burn. We have selected one particular case because the care encompassed so many of the newest elements of modern burn care, because it was such a dramatic injury, and because of the particular restrictions placed on the burn team by the patient's own wishes and religious beliefs.

A robustly healthy young man, 18 years old, was riding his restored Harley to work in a rural New England state. We will call him "Tim." A car suddenly backed out of a driveway and blocked his path. Tim swerved to miss the car, crashed into the mailbox, and slid, first with the bike and then under it, into a stone wall. The gas tank exploded. A passing motorist stopped and extinguished the flames with a garden hose before pulling the motorcycle off Tim. Although he was partially protected by his helmet, leather riding gloves, and work boots, the rest of his body suffered severe burns.

Tim was transported immediately by volunteer ambulance corps to the local hospital. His parents arrived while he was still awake and talking. Tim talked with the doctor on duty and his parents about his religious faith, his hopes for the future, and his wishes regarding his medical care. A Jehovah's Witness, Tim declared that while he wanted full and complete medical care, it could not include the transfusion of blood or blood products. He signed papers to that effect. Intravenous lines were inserted and his resuscitation with lactated Ringer's solution began. As arrangements for his transfer to the regional trauma center were being made, he developed respiratory difficulty that required intubation; a ventilator began to breath for him. He was transferred by helicopter to a medical center where burn physicians began his care. He received debridement and escharotomies (the cutting open of dead skin) to aid assessment of unburned tissue below and to allow swelling without compromising blood supply. The burn team understood his religious preference against therapeutic use of blood and would honor it, even though they did not agree with his decision; he would, most likely, die without new blood. His care seemed futile, a senseless prolongation of a life that essentially ended when the gas tank exploded. The family, while strongly believing in God's will, nonetheless wished his intensive medical care to proceed within such limitations.

Calls were made to several burn centers currently doing research on artificial skin, cultured skin, and other techniques that might help such a severely burned adult. After several declined to accept the transfer because of the proscription against blood, a center over 1,000 miles away agreed to accept him. Tim was transferred by ambulance to the airport, flown by private jet to New York, and then by helicopter to the receiving hospital. He was now five days post-injury. His organs were all functioning well except that he still required artificial ventilation. There was no evidence of infection, yet. The only significant finding, other than the severe burn, was a red cell count (hematocrit) of 18 instead of a normal 36. This count was still sufficient for oxygen delivery but dangerously low for surgery, and removal of the burn wound by surgery was essential to his survival. Such surgery typically requires many units (pints) of transfused blood. His care was at a crossroads. No surgery, and he would certainly die. If the wound was not closed—first with temporary skin grafts from pigs or cadavers, or with some other artificial skin substitute—infection was inevitable. But even if all the burn wound was successfully removed and temporary coverage occurred, there was insufficient healthy skin on his body for the final step, grafts of his own skin.

The problems presented by his care were multiple. Paradoxically, each one was potentially solvable by itself, but in the aggregate they seemed insurmountable. Nonetheless, the team conferred and agreed to a strategy that identified each barrier, applied a solution, and still managed to honor the patient's and his family's wishes.

Techniques Available for Tim's Care

The burn team needed to treat the following areas: fluid replacement, skin, blood, infections, and nutrition. As we describe Tim's case further, we will discuss these in turn throughout this chapter.

Fluid Replacement

When a burn wound is large, early death has come, historically, from the loss of body fluids. The pioneering studies of Underhill, then those of Harkins, Cope, and Moore, led to various formulas for fluid replacement. The initial treatment Tim received included the infusion of large volumes of lactated Ringer's solution. The formula for calculating his fluid requirement is based on his weight and the extent of his burn with adjustments based on his response (urine output, vital signs, cardiac function, etc.). One commonly used formula, refined by Dr. Charles Baxter, is the Parkland formula. Baxter was one of the young physicians working in Boston at the time of the Co-coanut Grove fire. This formula, although commonly used in the U.S., is not used world-wide. For example, in the "undeveloped" world—except for some western-style medical facilities—fluid replacement is done principally by oral hydration with a saltwater solution. In England, large quantities of plasma are given during the first phases of burn care. In central Europe, exchange transfusions—removing the patient's blood, while infusing fresh donor blood—is the preferred method of resuscitation. All these methods are effective in maintaining the intravascular volume of blood and fluid needed to preserve organ function, deliver oxygen, and maintain vital signs. The Parkland formula (named for the hospital in Dallas where Dr. Baxter has been the director of the burn center for many years), calculates the amount of fluids required by burn patients for the first 24 hours after the injury, based on the weight of the patient and the total body surface area burned (weight in kilograms × percent TBSA burned × 4cc). This formula allows a quick estimate of fluid requirements for any given adult patient with any given burn size up to 50 percent TBSA; thus it permits safe resuscitation for the majority of burn victims during the first 24 hours after their injury.

In the first few days, the fluid leak causes a decrease in the levels of serum albumin, a substance important in maintaining plasma and blood within the vascular space. During this phase of resuscitation, the patient, who may have become grotesquely swollen, rapidly loses extra fluid through diuresis. Replacing albumin is an important part of this process. In Tim's case, the use of albumin (by IV infusion) was permitted, although some Jehovah's Witnesses interpret that treatment as a use of blood.

The dilution of Tim's blood by the fluid resuscitation and the loss of red cells damaged during his burn injury resulted in a loss of 50 percent of his normal red cell mass. In the absence of the ability to give Tim blood, methods were employed to increase his own ability to make the red blood cells. He was given a "loading dose" of intravenous iron, and was started on a product of genetic recombination known as EPO-erythropoeitin (Epogen ®). Tim was one of the first non-renal patients to be treated with this substance. It worked well, as measured by his reticulocyte count — the means of assessing red cell production. He also continued to receive regular iron injections and vitamin supplements intended to stimulate red cell production.

Skin

Dead skin must be removed from the wounds, which must then be covered by something else to reduce the risk of fatal infection. We will discuss the removal of dead skin first, although both processes now often occur in the same operation, thanks to the dermatome. Debridement (that is removal) is usually part of the initial assessment of a patient; nurses, doctors, or burn technicians pick away dead skin with a forceps. Another method — under total anesthesia — is a scraping or shaving and scrubbing of the patient. Another method is "tanking": the patient is soaked in a Hubbard tank filled with water and a weak chlorine solution, then raised on a metal carrier for debridement. Since advances in pain care have not kept pace with this method of debridement, it has been replaced with formal surgical debridement under anesthesia at most centers.

Once the dead tissue is removed, coverage of the wound becomes the top priority. Studies by Burke at Harvard have shown that the risk of mortality declines in proportion to the decrease in the size of the burn wound as skin coverage is obtained (1976). Naturally the material used to cover is very important. The choices include the following: autograft (the patients own skin), homograft (skin from other humans, either cadaver skin or the skin of a living relative; best of all is the skin of an identical twin), heterograft (skin from another species, usually pig), artificial skin, or cultured skin. The temporary substitutes may buy time for the patient while efforts to obtain permanent skin coverage are underway, either by artificially culturing the patient's own skin in a laboratory, or by permitting existing donor sites in the patient to heal so they can be re-harvested. Harvesting is typically done with an electric dermatome.

The single most important surgical advance in burn care came from a surgeon working independently in the former Yugoslavia. Dr. A. Zora Janzekovic found a way to remove dead skin and to graft over the wound in one operation. When she presented her work (2,615 burn patients, 1,345 of which were children, with no deaths) at an international burns symposium in 1975, the effect was electric and her method was immediately recognized as a singular and spectacular leap forward (Heimbach 1987). She had taken the technique ordinarily used to harvest donor skin and adapted it to the slicing off of the burn wound itself, down to its lowest layer, still preserving vital tissues immediately below. This "tangential excision," when applied to moderate to deep partial thickness wounds, permits the grafting of burns during the same operation. Since this removal can be done 24–48 hours after the actual burn event — or once the patient has been stabilized — it is called "early excision."

Janzekovic's technique also benefited from a technique developed by Tanner. Harvested donor skin is cut with a series of parallel slits (see Figure 21), then pulled from the sides to expand the skin into a mesh with diamond spaces; this expansion permits 1, 3, 6 or even 9 times the area of the original harvest to cover the burn wound (see Figure 22). Janzekovic's detailed studies demonstrated that such excision and grafting resulted in quick healing, less scarring and shorter hospital stays, and could be equally effective on burns of 10 or 40 percent TBSA. Preserved elements of dermis, if left in contact with burned tissue often undergo a delayed transformation into dead tissues; her approach reduced such conversion and reduced subsequent burn infection risks. Comparison of survival statistics (such as complication rates and length of stay) from several burn centers indicates that significant improvements in outcome result from the aggressive, early surgical burn wound management (Feller 1980) — which Janzekovic's technique, often in combination with Tanner's meshed skin, allows.

Using a biological dressing immediately as the burn itself is excised is not a new or modern idea. The first written account of biological dressing occurs in the Ebers Papyrus (1500 B.C.E.), which recommends an application of meat, honey, and a warm oiled frog (!) applied to an open wound to stimulate healing (Robson et al. 1973). Subsequent references were equally colorful, though of questionable therapeutic value. Paracelsus wrote of a burn salve consisting of fat from old hogs and bears, roasted angleworms scraped from the skull of a hanged man, dried brain, and even a portion of a genuine mummy (Pack and Davis 1930). Peters lists the large number of heterografts (skin from different species) recommended between 1682, when Canaday advocated water lizards, and today, when pig skin is used. Use of heterografts was slowed by social attitudes, such as religious injunctions against skin substitutes during the seventeenth and eighteenth centuries and antivivisection laws in the 1890s.

The use of homografts (skin from human donors) was advocated during Renaissance Italy when slaves' noses were used to replace those of the upper class men lost during duels. These homografts were widely reported as successful, but the long-term results — which must have been disastrous — were

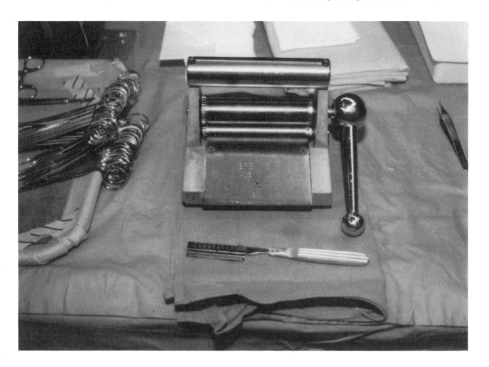

Figure 21. Skin mesher and knife. The skin mesher allows the expansion of harvested skin in ratios ranging from 1.5/1 to 9/1, increasing the ability of a little skin to cover a big wound. The skin when expanded develops a diamond-like net pattern that may or may not fade as healing progresses. The "Goulian" knife is a hand-held dermatome frequently used for debridement and occasionally for harvesting skin. Photo by Jane Arbuckle Petro.

ignored (Gibson). The first known application of homograft skin to a burn was by Pollock in 1870. These and subsequent attempts to close the burn wound permanently with skin from a source other than the patient were doomed to failure because rejection occurs as the host's immune system recognizes the antigens in the skin as "foreign." During World War I physicians attempted to "fix" the burned skin with picric acid (or, during the following decade, with tannic acid) into a kind of leather that would cover the wound; this approach recognized the value of a "biological" dressing but had no long-term advantages. During World War II attempts at temporary wound closure included using a mixture of titanium dioxide, lanolin, Vaseline, castor oil, beeswax, and sulfanilamide. Brown and McDowell began to use homografts as temporary wound covers, an application that was both safe and effective, leading the way for the management of very large burns. Brown and his co-workers later showed how the use of these grafts as dress-

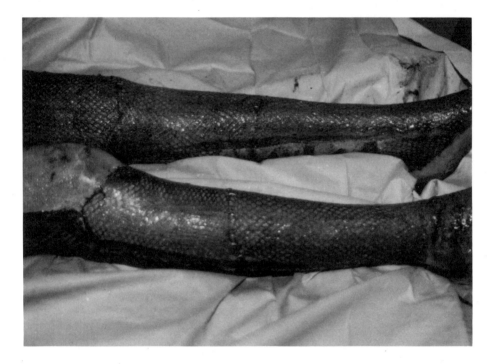

Figure 22. Legs covered by meshed and other grafts. This patient suffered extensive burns to the lower legs. The most obvious grafts are the 3/1 meshed grafts identifiable by their small diamonds, but there are also sheet grafts (on the right knee); staples help hold them in place. Photo by Jane Arbuckle Petro.

ings could prepare the wound for eventual coverage with skin taken from the patient (Peters 1980); common sites — obviously unburned — included stomach, back, and thighs.

Heterografting (also referred to as xenografting) regained popularity as a temporary wound cover in 1957 when Silvetti reintroduced the idea suggesting the use of bovine embryonic skin. The use of pig skin ("porcine heterograft") was popularized because of convenience and widespread availability from the successful sausage industry. Only later was the relative biocompatibility between pig and human understood as an additional beneficial factor.

Non-biological skin replacement, such as synthetic material, provides a skin-like wound barrier that reduces evaporative water loss across the wound, decreases protein loss, and protects against bacterial or fungal invasion. These commercial products are quite useful: they provide effective short-term cover, have an extended shelf life with easy storage, can be sterile, and can be impregnated with antibiotics if necessary. Unless the wound is partial thickness and will heal itself, these products can only be useful if there is a "real" skin cover available soon.

During the 1960s burn units began to harvest and store cadaver and donor skin for use as temporary burn cover. The skin excised during reduction mammoplasty or abdominoplasty would be saved and frozen for later use. These small pieces were useful in small burns, and as an aid in preparing chronic open wounds for closure. Cadaver donors were also used; while alive, these persons had given full consent. Long strips of skin could be harvested using standard dermatome techniques. While working in a burn unit in New York City one of us (JAP) collected skin by this method. Residents and medical students working on the burn service were also responsible for performing this somewhat gruesome task. Very few members of the burn team refused to participate in the harvesting as everyone recognized the great value of the donated skin, and were grateful for the precious gift. Amniotic membranes were also harvested from placentas in the delivery room and used as biological dressings, especially for partial thickness scald burns in children. These reduced the risk of infection, protected the wound as it was healing, and eliminated the need for painful dressing changes.

As fear of blood-borne infection became a concern in the late 1970s (even before AIDS), regulation of this process and expensive testing procedures reduced the number of facilities equipped to harvest cadaver skin, which is now an expensive and sought-after commodity. The use of amniotic membranes was similarly abandoned in the developed world. The ready availability and low cost of amniotic membranes still make them attractive in many burn centers, but the use of such alternative biological dressings carries too high a risk of infectious disease. The search for inexpensive, safe alternatives continues.

The luxury of expensive replacements does not exist in many areas of the world. In central Brazil, for example, human skin is often obtained from living donors of the burn patient's family. This same center also experiments with frog skin as a cheaper alternative to pig skin and reports good results. The facility has little financial support (compared to those in the United States), while treating a huge number of patients, some 10,000 to 12,000 per year, versus fewer than 1,000 per year even in the largest centers in the United States.

In India, Subrahmanyam (1994) reported on the use of honey-impregnated gauze compared to amniotic membranes in the treatment of partial thickness burns. Although the pain relief of the amniotic membrane was judged to be superior, the honey-treated group had the fewest infections and healed much more rapidly. The return to remedies of other eras—typically cheap, readily available, and efficacious—is not yet apparent in the U.S., but, as cost effective measures are increasingly applied, such treatments will likely be investigated.

One of the more recent, expensive, and dramatic developments in the

United States is skin culturing. A small piece of a patient's skin is harvested, disintegrated to clumps of cells, then grown on a sterile matrix to produce a large piece of skin — a variety of autograft. This technique was perfected by Rheinwald, Green, and their colleagues at Harvard Medical School. The possibility of using this technique in a clinical setting was described by Green and Kehinde as early as 1979. O'Connor and Milliken et al. proposed using the technique in large burns (1981), and it was subsequently used by Gallico and his colleagues in the treatment of two young brothers at the Shrine Burns Institute in Boston in 1984. Both brothers had full-thickness burns involving 90 percent TBSA, but they were treated successfully. Green's technique, when perfected, led to the creation of a commercial venture, which offers cultured skin as part of the new emerging biotechnology market. A sample of skin, harvested from a massively burned patient, could be grown into several square meters of cultured epidermis within three weeks. The limits of this technique include the length of time from injury to the product's availability and the production of only epidermis, not dermis as well. (Both elements are essential for full skin function and for skin durability.) There is also a prolonged time when the cultured epidermal cells are extremely fragile, even when in place upon the patient, and the cosmetic result, while not bad, is not fully satisfactory.

Newer technology includes the use of a collagen matrix as dermis and cultured epidermis, or of allogenic (not containing the antigens which lead to rejection) cultured skin (cultured foreskin, actually), which can be grown and stored for long periods of time. As of this writing, these techniques are in clinical trials in the United States and should be available for general use before the end of the 1990s. Cultured foreskin is already available in Australia, where it has been in use for several years. Although not available at the time of Tim's injury, this product permits application of the skin at the time of burn wound excision, thus eliminating one stage in the series of operations. It also finds application in other conditions. In fact, cultured foreskin was pioneered by a dermatologist in Australia, whose children had a condition known as epidemolysis bullosa congenita (EBC), a genetic condition in which the outer layer of the skin, the epidermis, cannot maintain its attachment to the underlying layer, the dermis. The repeated trauma of normal activities leads to the loss of the fingernails within the first few months of life, and the gradual loss of finger length and hand function, as well as open wounds at other sites of mild trauma, such as picking up the child by the underarms. Dr. Mark Eisenberg developed the cultured foreskin as a means of grafting these frequently occurring wounds, reducing pain and scarring. His patented technique is now being tested in the United States as a method for burn care as well as a treatment for EBC.

The increasing proliferation of cultured skin companies indicates not just the widespread interest in burns, but an interest in wounds themselves as investment opportunities. The proliferation of wound care centers in the

United States similar to that of commercial hospitals, cancer treatment centers, AIDS treatment programs, and diabetes centers, indicates the commercial viability of these disease-specific enterprises. Some investors have estimated that there may be as many as 4 million Americans who have chronic, non-healing wounds that could benefit from cultured skin grafts (Beard, 1994). Thus burns, although the most dramatic application, represent a relatively small part of the potential market. Skin culturing is, in theory, relatively simple: skin has uniform cell type with a definable but limited function. The commercial culturing of other tissues and complex organs — kidneys, heart, bone, nerve, liver, pancreas, and so on — may eventually be possible.

Treatment of Tim's Case

Thus a complex array of techniques and technology could be applied to Tim's case. The small areas for available autograft (self grafting) could be harvested and meshed to cover critical areas such as the neck, hands, and arms. Areas of less deep injury could be excised and covered with cadaver skin. A few square centimeters of his skin were sent to a lab for the creation of his own cultured epithelium.

Frozen cadaver skin was ordered from the skin banks at Cornell and Yale. Since this covering is temporary, it can be taken from persons of differing races. Some patients have had stripes of black and white skin, allowing for jokes about looking like a zebra. Some even have had temporary tattoos, a legacy from a cadaver.

The excision of Tim's burn wounds proceeded region by region, with a team of anesthesiologists and surgeons focusing on losing as little blood as possible. In order to accomplish those dual goals, the anesthesia plan was to maintain a low, stable blood pressure, just enough to permit perfusion of the essential organs (brain, heart, and kidneys) but minimizing flow to the skin. The surgery used an old fluid-replacement technique called clysis, in which large volumes of fluid containing diluted epinephrine are injected under the skin in order to constrict blood vessels. The excision of the burn wound in most areas proceeded to the level of the fascia, just above muscle. Areas of slightly less severe burn were excised tangentially. The trunk, then each extremity was excised using these methods. The process took several days, with loss of less than a cup of blood each time. The resulting open wound was covered with cadaver skin, pending arrival of cultured skin.

Another method of wound debridement, a "natural" one was also considered and attempted. The time interval between each surgery left Tim at considerable and constant risk of infection; in order to speed the debridement and reduce the number of surgeries, maggot therapy was attempted. The blowfly, a common species related to the house fly, can inhabit human wounds in its larval stage. While a surgical resident, one of the authors (JAP) had known several patients who came out of the mountains of Kentucky with large leg ulcers or advanced cancers inhabited by these larval forms. As repulsive as it seemed, they played an important role by eating away the dead flesh of the wound but not harming the intact tissues surrounding it. They probably also produced locally effective antibiotics, reducing risk for infection.

The entomology department of the Natural History Museum in New York City has been studying larval infestations of human wounds (sometimes seen in city hospitals) and provided the address of a fishing supply company in Alabama which cultivated blowfly larva. Several containers were shipped by overnight express. With the hospital's full knowledge of the risks—the larvae could transmit infection or they could mature and infest the burn center; even the possibility of negative publicity—plus the agreement of the family and the patient, the maggots were applied to the undebrided burn wounds. Whether the burn wound was too dry or the Silvadene cream was distasteful to them, the maggots failed to show any interest in feeding on dead tissue. After two days of spirited effort (and some revulsion), they were removed. Maggots are used in other burn centers, but such use is not widely acknowledged. Even burn care workers harbor certain taboos!

Blood

The use of blood and blood products (plasma, platelets, red blood cells) has been a driving force in the advance of increasingly bold and invasive surgical procedures. Blood banks and blood drives originated from the need for safe, high volumes of blood during World War II and later for the accidents of civilian life. The blood industry in the United States includes powerful for-profit and not-for-profit industry sectors.

The Jehovah's Witness movement, a conservative Protestant sect started in the 1940s, is deeply opposed to the use of blood among their members, believing that to receive a blood transfusion prevents an individual's entry into heaven. This injunction is based on several biblical passages: "Only flesh with its soul—its blood—you must not eat" (Gen. 9: 3, 4). "Be firmly resolved not to eat the blood" and "You must not eat it in order that it may go well with you and your sons after you" (Deut. 12: 23, 25). The challenge of the Witnesses (and others) has led the medical profession to examine blood usage carefully and to create blood substitutes that can change and improve common standards of care. A most striking example is the shift, in cardiac surgery, from priming the open heart pump with large quantities of human blood—as was done until the mid-1980s—to priming it with saline solutions, and then using autologous donor blood (given by the patient) if necessary. Witnesses oppose the use even of autologous blood. In a surprising result, their post-operative cardiac care has shown that low blood levels are better tolerated than previously believed and, in fact, the post-cardiac surgery patient may even do better with "thin" (diluted) blood, which has a lower viscosity.

The use of autologous transfusion, which involves saving one's own blood in anticipation of scheduled surgery, became even more widespread following the scandal over AIDS transmission through donated blood in the early and mid-1980s. Current blood banking practices continue to be negatively affected, with a marked decline in the donor pool and persistent suspicion over blood safety among both the lay public and the medical profession. Burn care, however, generally demands that large volumes of blood be available and used. Red cells, essential for oxygen delivery, are damaged as they pass through the tissues of the burn wound or are burned themselves at the time of injury, resulting in a dramatic drop in blood count in the days following a major burn such as Tim's. In 1961 Topley used radioactive isotope methods to demonstrate a 20–40 percent loss of red cell mass during the shock phase of injury (first 48 hours). In addition to the blood lost at the time of injury, the very treatment of burns (lab tests and dressing changes, for example) can result in substantial blood losses, especially over days and weeks.

In order to reduce the effects of this blood loss, several measures were taken to conserve Tim's precious red cells. Besides the careful surgery and efforts to shore up his red cell production, laboratory tests were kept to a minimum and the samples were collected as if he were a "premie," taking tiny amounts and using more expensive lab methods. Even so, Tim's blood count dropped slowly and steadily: 18, 14, 13, 12, 10, and stayed around 10 for the first three weeks of his hospital care. Although decreased by the reduced amount of red cell carrying capacity, his oxygen delivery (measured by pulse oximeter) remained high: 98 percent. If the oxygen delivery dropped enough, his cadaver skin grafts would not "take" and when the cultured skin arrived, his wounds would not be adequately prepared for them.

As his condition stabilized and then improved, it became possible to extubate Tim and remove him from the ventilator. Once he was breathing independently, we could consider another means of maintaining oxygen levels in his tissue. Once or twice a day, he was placed in a hyperbaric chamber large enough to hold one person and pressurized to 2.5 atmospheres in a pure oxygen environment. The supersaturation of his blood and all other tissues remained effective for up to 6 hours after each 90-minute treatment. The use of hyperbaric oxygen in burn treatment is still classified as experimental, despite clinical research indicating its efficacy in speeding healing and reducing hospital stay in moderate to severe burns (Cianci 1994, Niu et al. 1987) and its usefulness in treating certain types of infections (Knighton 1984).

The search for a safe, cost-effective, and easily stored artificial blood substitute for use by Jehovah's Witnesses has led to the development of a substance called Fluosol. Available for limited uses, it was approved by the FDA for application in Tim's case on a "compassionate relief" protocol. In the later stages of his care and during surgery, it was used twice for blood replacement. During the most critical stages of care, when Tim became septic, profoundly anemic (hematocrit less than 10), and in shock, Fluosol and a number of other interventions were applied. The actual source of his recovery from each episode was probably his excellent physical condition at the time of the accident.

Infections

The course of infections found in the burn patient parallels the history of human bacterial infections and hospital-acquired infectious illness. These infections can stem from many sources. Burn patients hospitalized in the 19th century were kept in general wards where they succumbed to the common agents of death, *Staphylococci* and *Streptococci*. Common in nature, these bacteria often came to the patient, ironically, on the hands and clothes of the physicians and nurses providing his or her care. Semmelweiss first noted that physicians and medical students performing autopsies prior to making rounds in the maternity ward caused a higher maternal mortality from puerperal sepsis than was found on those wards where the doctors did not do autopsies. In 1875, Lister (without knowing initially of Semmelweiss's work, but using Pasteur's descriptions) demonstrated that wound infections could be prevented if "anti-septic" techniques were applied. His procedures — use of carbolic acid sprays and washes — significantly reduced the incidence of hospital-acquired (nosocomial) infections. Later, the introduction of rubber gloves reduced the incidence of death among physicians — who had also succumbed to the infections they often transmitted — as well as further reducing infections transmitted from physician to patient.

In 1934 J. Dunbar reviewed the cases of burns treated at the Glasgow Royal infirmary during the preceding 100 years, paying special attention to the problems of infections seen there. He observed that, using modern culture techniques, it was possible to show that burn wounds were sterile at the time of admission, that is, had no identifiable bacteria present, but that within 12 hours 80 percent of the patients had positive *Streptococcus* cultures. D. M. Jackson, in a 1991 article, recalled the care given to a patient with a 20 percent burn who had been admitted to a surgical ward in 1939. It was actually against the rules to admit such a patient to the surgical ward so the patient was temporarily transferred to — of all places — the septic ward, where carbuncles (skin infections) and ischiorectal abscesses (infections of the anus) were treated, until another hospital would admit such a patient. Even the most meticulous surgical care in sterile operating rooms — with all attendants carefully gloved and masked — can infect a burn wound. Although a healthy patient with a small wound will rarely get an infection, large burn wounds cause a generalized decrease in immune function that makes infection nearly inevitable.

A large open wound coupled with an impaired immune response provides a natural target for bacterial invasion. The patient's own intestinal flora provide a rich source of bacteria for that wound infection through a process called translocation. This occurs during shock or after a few days with no oral caloric intake; bacteria from inside the large intestine can migrate through the mucosal barrier, enter the blood stream, and travel to the burn wound or to the lungs, causing pneumonia. After the introduction of intravenous fluid therapy and the reduction of burn deaths from shock in the acute phase, infection became the commonest cause of delayed burn death, occurring in the weeks that followed the original injury. This risk prevailed until the development of a safe, effective topical burn cream, and the use of improved nutrition support that was essential to ward off infection.

The search for the perfect burn salve to prevent infection and promote healing continued after World War II. Most of the substances applied to the burn wound described in the previous chapter did little, if anything, to prevent infection, except those that contained wine, honey, or copper sulfate. The discovery of the sulfonamides and penicillin were hailed as potential topical wound agents that would control burn wound infections. Regrettably, clinical trials in the 1940s, including the experience at the Cocoanut Grove, showed that these substances had little if any effect on wound management or even burn outcomes. Other early antibiotics showed efficacy against staphylococcal and streptococcal skin flora, but these both quickly developed resistance to the new antibiotics and continued to infect burn wounds. Still other topical agents had the potential for harming the patient. The wound was a two-way avenue: fluid and protein leaking out, the substances applied leaking in — often to the detriment of the patient. Tannic acid, popularized by Davidson in 1926, was used extensively until the 1940s, when MacIndoe condemned it because of its side effects: both liver toxicity and deformities to the hands. MacIndoe preferred the use of saline soaks, which simultaneously softened and cleansed the burn wound, coupled with an "open" or "exposure" method, allowing the eschar to dry into a medium inhospitable for bacterial growth. The exposure method was strongly advocated by Blocker in the United States and Wallace in the United Kingdom. The opposite method, using a paraffin gauze bulky dressing, was equally strongly advocated by Allen and Koch (1942) in Chicago.

In Great Britain, collaboration between clinicians and Leonard Colebrook, a bacteriologist, lead to a search for an effective topical antibacterial which, like Prontosil, would control the burn wound flora. Colebrook first tried sulfanilamide cream but its initial promise faded as streptococcal bacteria became completely resistant to it by 1943. In that year penicillin became available but, as just noted, it proved ineffective. Though it protected against the gram positive organisms *Streptococcus* and *Staphylococcus*, it did not prevent the overgrowth of the wound by the gram negative organisms, predominantly *Pseudomonas*, an enteric (that is, from the gut) bacterium which rapidly replaced the gram positive organisms (staphylococcal or streptococcal) as the leading infectious agent of mortality.

Topical treatment with polymyxin cream was used in 1951 with some success as fewer gram positive organisms developed resistance, but *Pseudomonas* remained a serious problem. Through the 1950s and early '60s deafness, kidney damage, and the emergence of highly resistant organisms plagued topical therapies like polymixin, polybactrin powder, gentamycin and streptomycin. Then, in an attempt to better understand the pathophysiology of death following high velocity gunshot wounds (a phenomenon of war first apparent in the Korean conflict), Lindsay, at the Walter Reed Institute of Research, began an investigation of the efficacy of local antibiotics in massive muscle injuries in goats. He found that Sulfamylon® cream appeared to be highly effective in reducing infection in these complex wounds. Lindberg and Moyer, at the Surgical Research Unit at Brooke, tested the cream on a rat burn model and showed a dramatic reduction in mortality which, when tested on human burn wounds, also held true. Moncrief reported a reduction in mortality of patients with burns covering 30–60 percent TBSA from 60 percent before the use of Sulfamylon® to 26 percent after its introduction (Artz 1969).

In 1965 Carl Moyer introduced the use of 0.5 percent silver nitrate solution and showed 3 percent of patients so treated showed evidence of *Pseudomonas* infection as compared to 70 percent of patients treated with penicillin cream. The chief disadvantages of silver nitrate (the active ingredient in photographic emulsion) are the staining of all surfaces it touches — including skin, fabric, and tiles — and the need to use large bulky dressings which must be changed frequently. While both silver nitrate and Sulfamylon were effective, neither was ideal. In addition to the messiness of the silver nitrate, large burns treated with it developed complex toxicity of water and electrolytes. Sulfamylon caused changes in kidney function and, if the patient had an inhalation injury, as is often the case in big burns, increased the rate of pulmonary complications, and death.

The development of Silvadene® in 1968 represented a major advance in burn care. A combination of silver ion and sulfadiazene, it was developed at Columbia University by Dr. Charles L. Fox. The efficacy of the silver ion (there is little argument about its antibiotic action even today) and the broad spectrum coverage of the sulfonamides was designed to provide maximum protection against infection. This product, developed during the 1960s and introduced into clinical use in the early 1970s, has become the gold standard for topical burn care. Initially it was quite expensive and therefore used only in the developed world, where high pharmaceutical costs are accepted as part of patient care. The patent rights on it expired in the late 1980s, however, permitting generic production, cost reduction, and wider availability in many countries. Applied as a 10 percent cream, it has many advantages: it is painless on application to both full thickness and partial thickness wounds, is effective against both gram positive and gram negative organisms, is only rarely absorbed in high enough quantities to cause toxicity, and can be applied with an absorbent dressing, thus allowing better patient mobility and requiring dressing changes only once a day.

Tim's Treatment Continues

The initial wound treatment for Tim was Silvadene, which protected him adequately at first. But after 5 to 10 days Silvadene loses its efficacy as resistant organisms such as *Enterococcus, E. coli,* and other bacteria became predominant. With the onset of sepsis, first caused by pneumonia, then wound infection, systemic intravenous antibiotics were started. But even these have limitations. The early hopes that systemic antibiotics would prevent infection were shown to be groundless during the treatment of survivors of the Cocoanut Grove fire; equally disappointing were MacIndoe's experiences treating military burns, the definitive work of Moncrief and Rivera in 1958, and a large, randomized trial by Ortiz-Montaserrio in Mexico that showed no difference in outcome between burns treated with antibiotics and those not so treated.

Since no single approach prevailed in modern care, Tim's burn team chose among several therapeutic strategies. Systemic antibiotics were selected based on culture and sensitivity results obtained from sputum cultures, blood cultures, and wound cultures. The topical antibiotics were changed first to silver nitrate solution, then to diluted iodine solutions. Treatment was designed to protect the temporary cadaveric skin, but later, the grafted cultured epithelium limited the selection of topical agents. Additional systemic anti-infective support included the administration of an experimental immunoglobulin, also a recombinant-gene product specific for gram negative sepsis. This was flown in by helicopter from the manufacturer in Philadelphia at a time when both Tim's blood pressure and blood count were dangerously low. From all these strategies, something worked, and he improved again, only to develop a serious new infection—*Candida*—a common yeast-like fungus that usually follows gram negative sepsis in burn patients. A new round of anti-fungal drugs was begun. While working to control infections, the burn team also kept an eye on Tim's nutrition.

Nutrition

Nutrition is a critical factor in burn survival. Asked to list those changes in management of burn patients that have most affected their survival, most professionals would select aggressive wound management and nutrition as the two key elements. Adequate caloric replacement—calculated on the basis of a patient's burn size, body surface area, weight and age—requires a high protein intake as well as sufficient vitamins and trace minerals. Such support maintains a more effective immune system, reduces muscle wasting, improves physiologic reserve, and has been shown to increase survival, reduce morbidity, and decrease infection rates. Whether by voluntary intake or tube, supervised feeding begins within 24 hours of injury and continues to the day of discharge.

Tim's requirement, in excess of 6,000 calories per day, clearly required a tube. Once his burn wound was excised and covered with cadaver skin, a feeding jejunostomy was inserted through his abdominal wall, allowing continuous feeding.

As patients near discharge from the hospital, staff urge them to eat aggressively, even to "eat their way out of the unit" because much depends on their nutritional status. The burn unit nutritionist is an important member of the burn team.

Tim's Outcome

After 7 weeks, all of Tim's body had been grafted. He was awake, talking, and entering the slow process of recovery, first getting out of bed to a chair, then out of his room into the central nursing station, then walking. His family visited every day; they had moved into the local community and found work. Local Jehovah's Witnesses provided them with an apartment near the hospital. Everyone began to talk about Tim's transfer back to the original treating hospital, and arrangements were made for it. His wounds, however, were very fragile and his hematocrit remained extremely low, staying around 13 and 14, about one-third the normal amount. But he was healed, could use his hands, walk, and function with increasing independence.

Two days before his transfer, while showering Tim suddenly complained of chest pain and passed out. His breathing stopped. He was re-intubated (his tracheotomy had not yet closed off) and resuscitated. Tests showed that he had had a pulmonary embolus. Despite the fact that his loss of consciousness was witnessed and oxygen and supportive therapy were initiated immediately, Tim remained on a ventilator, unconscious but with evidence of some brain activity, for several more weeks. While he was in the operating room for a minor surgical procedure on his abdominal jejunostomy tube, his heart suddenly stopped and could not be restarted. He had been in the hospital for almost four months and had nearly gone home. His burn wounds had healed, but he did not survive.

The team caring for Tim had included the plastic surgeons in charge of the burn center, specialists from infectious diseases, pulmonary medicine, hematology, anesthesiology, neurology, rehabilitation medicine, uncounted residents, interns and medical students, a superb assortment of nurses, burn technicians, respiratory therapists, technicians, x-ray technicians, pharmacists, even the hospital administrators. Outside the immediate hospital community, the drug representatives of the Fluosol manufacturer, the nurse practitioner from the cultured skin company, Biotech, and many neighbors and community representatives had all been invested in his outcome.

This death, while heartbreaking and discouraging, provided evidence that the nearly successful effort was worthwhile and that addressing each problem from a multi-disciplinary approach can provide a wide range of possible solutions for future patients, even while respecting patient wishes that restrict options. All burn surgery, for example, can be carried out with some reduction of blood loss. All laboratory studies can be evaluated more carefully, reducing the frequency and number of tests. There are indeed a lot of "neat things we can do," and a loss one time may make possible a win another time — to use over-simple terms. Within the larger community of the hospital, other services became interested in serving the Jehovah's Witness community and began to offer "bloodless" care. In an era where blood, despite careful screening, testing, and judicious administration can still be a source of hepatitis, transfusion reactions, and (rarely) AIDS, the approach of the Witnesses now seems more rational and reasonable than ever before.

Rehabilitation

Where do people go after they leave the burn center? What kind of rehabilitation do they need? What do they get? Given the sophisticated and intense care of the burn center, it would make much sense to have appropriate continuity of care following discharge. Regrettably this is typically *not* the case. Far less time, money, and attention is paid to the sequelae of burn injury, despite its profound importance for patients with large burns. In this section we will discuss the second challenge of modern burn care, the restoration of patients' pre-burn capacities.

Of the now thousands of published articles on burn rehabilitation appearing in the literature, 90 percent of them still focus on the rehabilitation that occurs *during* the initial hospitalization. The majority of the rest concern those patients who return to burn centers for some form of reconstructive surgery, leaving scant attention to other rehab issues. Another indication of neglect in this area is the tardy attention of the Social Security Administration, which only recently developed criteria for disability that applied to burn patients. Further, funding for rehabilitation research only recently became available and it faces an uncertain future at National Institutes of Health under current federal budget conditions.

Where Do Burn Patients Go After Hospitalization? The Case of Jeff

Jeff was a 23-year-old maintenance engineer for a large manufacturing plant. His job was to keep the building's heating and cooling systems working properly. While crawling along a tunnel to examine one of the pipes for a leak, he reached the site of the leak just as a co-worker, by remote control, turned a valve that sent through the pipe a powerful surge of superheated steam. The pipe ruptured and the steam blasted Jeff directly in the face. He was burned over about 20 percent of his body, all of it on his head, face, neck, arms, and hands. Alarms in the conduit tunnel alerted the plant foreman of an accident; even before Jeff backed out of the tunnel, emergency services had been notified. A helicopter delivered Jeff to the burn center within 25 minutes of the accident.

Steam is notoriously dangerous, whether in industry or from the radiator of a car—the source of many scald burns. Pressurized steam can attain and hold much greater temperatures than boiling water and in high volumes it will not cool rapidly enough to avoid serious burns. Jeff's injuries lacked the charred or blackened appearance of fire-caused third-degree burns, but the damage inflicted was just as severe. Because the blast was directed at his face and in a confined space, he was forced to breathe the superheated steaming air, causing deep thermal burns of his pharynx, larynx, and tracheobronchial tree. The rapid swelling of his burned face and airway required intubation by the emergency rescue team at the plant site. Without that intervention, he would have been dead on arrival.

Survival, however, was not guaranteed by this prompt action nor by his swift transportation to the burn center. During the following weeks, the damage to his lungs—which was far greater than the damage to his skin—contributed to severe pneumonia and multiple episodes of near strangulation as the lining of his trachea sloughed off, blocking his airway. Frequent bronchoscopy (direct visualization of his lungs with fiberoptic equipment) allowed for the removal of debris and pus and promoted the healing of his injured interior. His face, neck, arms, and hands were grafted, and once his neck was sufficiently healed, a tracheotomy was done so the injured larynx could also heal without the irritation and damage of a tube going from his mouth to his lungs. The shorter passage via the tracheotomy also made easier his "pulmonary toilet" (regular cleaning of his lungs by a respiratory therapist).

For several weeks, the severity of his illness left Jeff relatively unconscious, suffering burn delirium in addition to the effects of the heavy pain and sedative medications prescribed to keep him breathing properly, i.e., letting the machine do it for him. Gradually, Jeff's lungs began to heal and he was weaned from his ventilator. His level of consciousness increased, narcotics and sedatives were withdrawn, and he awoke. Now his progress accelerated: he got out of bed, ate, and, finally, talked. All of his burns had been grafted while he slept.

Now, his care centered on getting a full range of motion and strength back in his hands, arms, and legs, getting his tracheotomy removed, and fashioning the mask and Jobst garments he would have to wear for the next several months to reshape scars and prevent contracture, deformity, and disability. In these activities the occupational therapist and the physical therapist took the lead.

Although Jeff lived independently with his girlfriend for several months before his accident, his mother wanted him to return home for continued care after his discharge. Neither Jeff or the burn team agreed because the mother lived quite far away. But Jeff's girlfriend—worn out from the stress of the burn event and the treatment—disappeared. So, when discharge time came, friends picked him up for the long ride to his mother's. The staff were not surprised or very concerned when Jeff failed to keep his follow-up visit: such misses are common. Nonetheless, after he missed the next visit, the burn unit contacted his mother. Jeff had never arrived at her house.

The failure of burn patients to maintain contact with their treating physicians and staff is a chronic problem in the burn world. There are a number of factors that contribute to such poor follow-up. Like Jeff, many patients come from far away. Burn centers are regional services, often providing specialized care to an area of several hundred square miles. In New York City, for example, there were five burn centers in 1985 but only two in 1995. In New York State, burn centers in Albany and Syracuse closed between 1992 and 1995, leaving the center in Westchester, just north of New York, to cover burns for nearly half the state. In 1995, the burn center in Burlington, Vermont also closed, sending still more patients to Westchester, Boston, and even Canada. Such facilities are often a driving distance of three or more hours for these patients (many of whom cannot drive when released from the hospital). Long term follow-up studies of burn patients frequently report on fewer than 25 percent of all the patients discharged. As Roger Salisbury pointed out in his presidential address to the American Burn Association in 1993: "It certainly would strike politicians, lawmakers, laymen, and other physicians as somewhat bizarre that we are capable of sophisticated studies that result in culturing of skin in a laboratory but that we are unable to follow up our patients once they leave the hospital."

Jeff showed up at the unit three months later. He was terribly scarred, extremely short of breath, and so hoarse that he could not be understood when he talked. Within two hours of appearing in the office waiting room, he was admitted to the hospital, taken to the operating room, and had an emergency tracheotomy performed. The burn of his larynx, like that of his face and hands, had contracted, cutting his airway to almost nothing. Later, Jeff explained that he thought his mask was making him hoarse so he stopped wearing it after 10 days. He went off with his friends, binge drinking and traveling. When he returned to the area, he avoided the hospital because he thought the team would be mad at him for not wearing the mask. His reconstruction began during the second hospitalization: surgery to his face, hands, and larynx. The complex nature of that laryngeal injury alone would require several staged procedures that could only be done at yet another hospital thirty miles away.

Very few people could have survived the type of burn Jeff received. His innate strengths of youth and health, and even perhaps his lack of fear and sophistication, provided the reserves he needed not only during his initial care, but during the interval between his first and second visits to the burn center. His future is uncertain, however, because he is unable to perform his original job. Further, he used his severance pay from his union to buy a "muscle" car. After several operations, he was able to care for himself, do those "acts of daily living" that some rehabilitation programs like to brag about, and he even looked much better. But his voice was not clear or strong, he still needed his tracheotomy, and his social network had shrunk considerably.

Despite the amount of effort that goes into the salvage of these patients, until recently little attention has been paid to their follow-up. Follow-up studies by major burns centers report the outcomes of only a small sample of their patients, and do not comment on the unanswered questionnaires, missed appointments, and lack of data on the majority of their discharged patients (Petro and Salzburg 1992). Where do they go and what do they do? Does failure to ask that question, and the seeming inability to answer it, say anything about burn care today? In 1984 Eyles and his co-workers demonstrated the methodological failings of long term follow-up research with burn survivors and developed a sound proposal for how such studies should be conducted; it was ignored in the subsequent literature. Even burn care-givers seem resigned to follow-up failure — despite seeing many of their efforts undone by patients. This sense of fatalism among care-givers could also be a negative factor in delivery of care.

What do we know so far about the problems faced by burn patients after survival and discharge? First, scarring is inevitable, and its treatment — to obtain maximum improvement — will take two to five years. Second, grafted skin does not sweat and does not grow hair (unless hair follicles have survived in the deep dermis, in partial thickness burns); it will itch unbearably for several years, and, if subjected to repeated trauma, can become malignant 20 or 30 years later. (How much of this is true of the cultured skin products is still not clear, but there is little reason to suppose that it will be significantly different.) Third, treatment following discharge should include use of compression dressings, such as Jobst garments, to reduce scars, as well as lubrication of this skin twice daily or more. Fourth, psychological counseling should be available, especially for post-traumatic stress syndrome. Fifth, in less than 10 percent of patients, readmission for reconstructive surgery will be necessary, notably when hands and face have been involved, or when a massive burn has caused contractures.

The conditions that accompany prolonged hospitalization — such as decreased strength and endurance, post-traumatic stress, sleeplessness, irritability, frustration over the change in appearance and physical abilities; lost time, wages, work; separation from family, co-workers, and friends — all these can contribute to *disability* while not resulting in actual *impairment*. The distinction between disability and impairment, the relative permanency of the conditions, and the relationship between them and the long term rehabilitation are as yet unexamined in a prospective manner. Nor are these concepts effectively distinguished in contemporary Social Security policy, through workman's compensation ratings, or in other ways that could contribute to understanding what services are beneficial for burn patients (Salisbury 1992).

While there is a large body of competent and comprehensive literature on burn care, the literature on burn recovery — on life after the burn center — does not approach the former in detail, depth, or applicable conclusions. A review of the patients qualifying for disability under Social Security — the most likely source of funding for burn rehabilitation — indicates that, for the years 1981, 1982, and 1983, a total of 362, 130, and 52 people respectively were granted coverage for burn-related disability. During each of those years, an estimated 6,000–7,000 should have been eligible, assuming a disability rate of 5 percent for the 50,000+ people surviving major burn injury annually (Helm 1992). Criteria for disability impairment developed by the Committee on Rehabilitation of the American Burn Association were not adopted by Social Security until 1993.

The current high cost of burn care may be worthwhile in terms of human lives saved, but we cannot show what quality of life has been restored. Although the American Burn Association has recognized the need for information and programs involving long-term burn rehabilitation and has established criteria for these programs (see Salisbury, 1992), funding for such activities presently does not exist. The excitement over bio-technical research has not extended to rehabilitation or to the assessment of the psychological and other human costs for burn survivors. It is hard to imagine, for example, the effect on the patient of the necessity to wear, in public, tight, unattractive garments covering hands and face, especially in the summertime. Burn doctors have had to provide some patients with a letter of explanation, indicating the medical necessity of the mask, because (as we saw in Chapter 6) a mask can symbolize a hidden and therefore suspect identity. One patient, a tall Jamaican with a terrible facial burn, was stopped by the police regularly while wearing his mask as he walked through an upper class neighborhood to his job as a gardener. Fortunately, most burn patients do not have severe facial burns, and scars of the commonest burn accidents can most frequently be hidden by clothing. But even these scars — from the spilled coffee on the shoulder or the flame burn on the calf — stigmatize the bearer and often in the survivors' own self-image.

Studies of the psychological outcomes of burns begins with the work of Frances MacGregor, a social worker affiliated with Cornell Medical Center in New York City. Her work, concentrating on facial disfigurement, is powerful and thoughtful, using a case analysis technique. A further development on the psychosocial aspects of burn wounds, especially the effects of facial disfigurement and body image distortions, was developed by Norman Bernstein, whose book, *Emotional Problems of the Facially Burned and Disfigured* (1976) remains the definitive analysis of the subject. Others—including Scheffield et al., Blakeney et al., Bowder and Feller, Prasad et al. have limited their work to retrospective evaluations of burn patient populations. Sheffield reviewed the records of 212 patients admitted to the Mayo Clinic between 1977 and 1982 with moderate to major burns. The paper does not comment on whether any of the patients were lost to follow-up, but notes noncompliance rate of 50 percent. Overall, the study shows that a small percentage of their patients (10–15 percent) exhibited psychiatric or physical problems, but the majority reported the burn as having a minimal effect on their lives. Blakeney followed his patients for 2 years; Bowder and Feller in a longer follow-up, noted that significant burn-related problems arouse 7–10 years after injury. And Cobb, in a review of 245 patients (only 13 percent of patients originally seen in the burn unit, he notes) observes no long-term reduction on quality of life for adults, but significant problems for children. Compared with a growing body of literature on burn treatment— literature that is scientifically sound, based on principles of good statistics, clinical trials, laboratory research, and careful observation of outcomes— the lack of literature on burn rehabilitation is striking and tragic.

It may be that, as in other fields of medicine, the powerful attraction and instant gratification of critical, hospital-based care—with its attendant financial rewards and focus on the drama of the rapidly changing physiologic condition of the patient—and the intellectual challenge of overcoming the predictable, yet stormy course of intensive care overshadows the challenges of excellent rehabilitation. Yet in recent years there has been a significant increase in facilities dedicated to other programs for rehabilitation; for example spinal cord injuries, head injuries, and cardiac and sports medicine. What distinguishes these problems from burns? In cardiac medicine, for instance, one of the distinctions is the social and economic class represented by those who have heart disease and can seek care. The heroism of open heart surgery is rapidly being superseded by the use of coronary angioplasty—a non-surgical, minimally invasive technique for repairing the heart—and by the emerging body of knowledge about preventive care in heart disease. Thus, corporate America has begun to place a high value on "heart health" and to emphasize the values of diet, fitness, and prevention. (Furthermore, reimbursement for such activities is now considered cost-effective, certainly in contrast to open-heart surgery.) Head injury and spinal cord patients are now offered full rehabilitation services in specialized care facilities; such support, although expensive, is generally covered under health insurance policies, even by Medicare and Medicaid. By contrast, the cost of Jobst garments for burn survivors is not covered under most insurance policies. For children with Medicaid, the approval for the garments often takes several months, a critical time for reducing scar formation. Donated funds in the burn center are often used to purchase these for the children. Also — very practically speaking — the best results occur when the garments are worn 23 hours per day, but the state will only approve the purchase of one garment; how's a parent supposed to launder and dry it?

There is a wonderful exception to the generally bleak outlook for burn rehabilitation: the burn camp. The development of medically specific summer programs for children first occurred in 1968 with the establishment of the "Three Track Ski Club," a program for children from the amputee clinic at the Children's Hospital in Denver. A burn camp for children first appeared in Denver in 1985, also related to the Children's Hospital, and was followed by the Jaycee Burn Center in Chapel Hill, N. C. By 1992, there were 18 such programs, 13 within the U.S., two in Canada and one each in New Zealand, Australia, and Belgium (Doctor 1992). Staff for the camps includes members of the hospital burn team, adult burn survivors, firefighters, professional camp personnel, and interns from related fields. In order to optimize the camp experience for all children, those with severe pre-morbid psychopathology or those whose response to their injury is extreme are not admitted (Doctor 1992). This therapeutic milieu is designed to encourage full participation, avoid ridicule, and promote recovery.

The advances in burn care since the 1950s have included the nutritional management of patients, the acute management of severe injuries, the control of infection, the relief of pain, the reduction of scar formation and deformities associated with scars, and in the use of the multi-disciplinary team approach to patient care. These steps have been a result of both planned and unplanned factors. The development of specialized medical units during World War I and their refinement in World War II trained a large number of bright, dedicated individuals, whose intellectual curiosity and creativity was stimulated by the high numbers of patients treated during those war years. Gilles, in England, is credited as the founding father of modern plastic surgery. His unit at the Queen's Hospital in Sidcup during the early part of the century, developed a collaborative effort of surgical, dental, and anesthesia specialists, established a standard of care, and achieved good functional and cosmetic results in treating burned aviators and sailors in World War I. This model was reapplied with excellent results during World War II to burns, facial wounds, and hand injuries (Stark 1975). The first burn center in the U.S. was established at the Medical College of Virginia in 1947. That same year, Brooke Army Hospital in San Antonio organized the U.S. Army Institute of Surgical Research, which was dedicated to burn research and the care of injured members of the armed services. Brooke continued its work with burns during the Korean and Viet Nam wars and remains the premier training and research center for adult burns (Dimick 1993). The surgeons trained at the Institute of Surgical Research at Brooke Army Hospital have gone on to become the leaders of the American Burn Association and the chiefs of burn centers throughout the U.S.

Special mention needs to be given to the Shriners who, in 1962, decided to support specialized burn centers for children. In 1966 such a unit was opened in Galveston, Texas, followed by one in Cincinnati in February, 1968, and in Boston at the end of 1968 (MacMillan, 1974). These units provide free care to the children hospitalized in their units, and free follow-up care until age 21. Their long-term assessment of outcomes, achieving 95 percent follow-up rate of the cases admitted, is the highest of any program evaluating rehabilitation results. In addition to medical care, these units are among the premier burn research centers in the world, and are completely funded by the Shriners. The three Shrine Burn Centers are responsible for nearly 30 percent of the research papers presented at the American Burn Association's annual meeting. The cost of these activities was estimated to be $28 million per year in 1974.

By 1992, there were 198 burn centers in the United States, providing 2,243 specialized beds that treated one third of all patients hospitalized for burns. This availability of high-tech care is being jeopardized in the 1990s by the increasing attention to cost cutting in health care. More burn units are closing than opening; the decline during the previous decade has resulted in the net loss of about 50 burn centers. This decline, we hasten to add, stems from financial pressures, not from any significant drop in numbers of severe burns. Despite the documented effectiveness of treatment given by specialized centers and the reduction in mortality, morbidity, and length of hospital stay such care ensures, the decline continues.

This review of modern burn care demonstrates the complexity of the burn injury and the wide variations in treatment available to promote healing and recovery. Unfortunately, the same level of funding, research, and enthusiasm that has refined hospital care for burn patients has not existed in the development of rehabilitation after discharge. Furthermore, cost containment in health care, a reduction in available research money, and marginalization of the burn patient through the closing of burn centers, make issues of prevention even more important (see Chapter 10).

Chapter Nine
Icarus Recovers (or Dies)
How High Can a Survivor Fly?

In this chapter we will discuss outcomes burn survivors may experience months and even years after their injuries. Our point of comparison will be the figure of Icarus, presented in Chapter 5 above, whose injury was not only fatal but determined. The fall of Icarus was inevitable, a result of the sun, gravity, and other inexorable physical powers, as well as the psychological imperatives of a young man aiming to "go the limit." This myth, we believe, became a negative model well into modern times for at least part of our understanding of severe burns: that burns were inevitably tragic and fatal. By this way of thinking, the persons who died were the lucky ones, since their suffering was short. The survivors were doomed to something worse, an existence as monsters for all to see, wounded and crippled both in body and in mind. No wonder the severe burn became, for many, "the worst thing that could happen to you."

Our thesis, however, is that burns need to be reconceived or reimaged in the light of modern burn care. We suggest, therefore, a rewriting of the myth of Icarus. Yes, some burn victims will plummet to their deaths even with the best of care — and we will speak of those first. But most — and especially those who receive modern care — will recover. They will recover in two senses: (1) recover meaning "to regain health" but also (2) re-cover, meaning "to have full covering of healthy skin once again." We may imagine Icarus as falling until a hand reaches out to catch him, to cradle him, to nurse and support him while he heals. Healing done, he (or she) may fly again. These new flights may have limits because of injuries, grafted skin, or a new wisdom about the body's limits, but Icarus, with proper care, flies again in the vast majority of cases.

The Minority of Burn Patients Who Die

It would be easy to write this book to extol all the superb medical techniques and to ignore the limitations. Clearly there are burn cases that medicine cannot "solve," and some burn patients will inevitably die. In the United States, an annual mortality rate of about 3 percent in a burn unit is typical. Of, say, 300 admissions in the course of year (an average number for a regional burn unit), some nine will die. Two major factors account for many of these deaths. First is the extent of the wound — 90 percent or more — with a lot of full thickness, and perhaps an inhalation injury or other injuries. Second is the health status of the patient: the very young, the elderly, and those with already poor health are much more likely to succumb to their injuries; combined factors — say, age and poor health — will given an even higher likelihood of death. Even before hospital care, some victims die at the scene of the accident from the severity of the burns, suffocation, electrical shock, or associated injuries, to the head, for example. (Such deaths, since they occur outside the burn unit are not reflected in burn unit data.) The geographical location of the accident can make a difference as well: a city-dweller might find paramedical help arriving in five minutes, whereas a person burned in a remote area might have to wait an hour or more for help to arrive. Even at the hospital, some injuries are beyond the abilities of medicine to heal, although palliative care may ease the patient's last hours.

For persons who arrive at the burn center, the odds of survival are much improved, especially if treatment in the field and in transport has been adequate during the so-called "golden hour," the first 60 minutes following the injury, when medical care makes a critical difference. In the field, paramedics must, by standard of care, initiate treatment no matter how futile it may appear. At the unit, however, burn personnel have some latitude in how aggressively to treat cases where treatment is clearly futile. Having discussed the treatment choices with the burn patient and/or family, the burn team may restrict its efforts to easing the suffering — but never, by current ethical and legal norms, to hastening death. In the most severe cases death typically occurs in 12 to 24 hours as organ systems fail. All burn deaths are cases for the medical examiner, who may choose whether to autopsy the body. Postmortem analysis sometimes reveals causes that can be rectified later so that other lives may be saved — for example, poisonous gases that fabrics in airplane interiors give off when on fire.

Deaths in the unit are generally unwelcome, because the staff's values are strongly for survival and recovery and because our culture in general is death-aversive. Sometimes frank discussion among the staff of the place death has in human life will help relieve unrealistic expectations. A medical outlook that fears death or sees death only as an implacable enemy will put stress on the staff unnecessarily: having a patient die should not automatically be construed as a failure. A psychiatrist or chaplain might talk with staff about how many cultures and religious traditions see a desirable state after death. For some caregivers — and some units in general — death is understood as a possible and sometimes even desirable outcome, especially when prospects for rehabilitation are very dim, for example in an elderly patient with crippling injuries. In some religious traditions, death is considered the highest flight of all, for example the symbolism of the butterfly at some Christian funerals to represent the metamorphosis from the chrysalis to a new and wonderful life. Mixing the traditions, we might say that Icarus, the former larva, bursts forth into beautiful flight beyond mortal life.

It is also important to speak sensitively with family and friends and to provide support in seeking out the patient's wishes for treatment. Are there any advance directives, such as a Living Will or a Health-Care Surrogate? It is important to maintain whatever patient autonomy is possible, especially when treatment, other than palliative care, is clearly futile. There are many complex issues here that we can only mention. Should a dying patient have an intensive care bed in the burn unit, especially if another patient who might live can use it? Should the unit's unvarying response be to treat aggressively? Should insurance or a hospital's endowment have to pay huge costs for futile treatment, especially if the burn was incurred during high-risk behaviors, such as smoking in bed, intoxication, or riding a motorcycle recklessly? These are difficult issues, and they are likely to continue to be present in burn units facing life-and-death situations.

How High Can a Survivor Fly?

Turning to the 97 (or so) percent who survive their burns, we can discuss two levels of their recovery, the physical level of tissues and biological functioning, and the wider contexts of healing on psychological, spiritual, and social levels. In each case we will divide them in three groups, keeping in mind that there is much individual variation. At one extreme, the patients leave with considerable problems, deficits, loss of limbs, functional impairments, sleep disorders, pain, itching scars, and more. At the other extreme some patients have after-effects for a while, but eventually return to virtually their pre-burn state. One of the large factors in outcome, of course, is the state of the patient at the time of the burn. A street person who took little care about diet and other health practices will typically have a slower healing course and a worse result than a healthy person.

"We Did the Best We Could"

The toughest cases leave with considerable damage: ears burned off, fingers or entire limbs amputated. Some patients are profoundly depressed. Electrical injuries are among the worst, mummifying a hand or even a limb. Not only is the outcome — upon leaving the hospital — hard on the patient and family and friends, but burn-care personnel often feel regret or even failure that, in the traditional phrase: "a better result could not be achieved."

In some cases, underlying conditions are still present or even worse: a patient arriving with illnesses such as diabetes or AIDS will also leave with them, and the burn staff will have the challenge of treating those entities along with the burn itself. In other cases, the burn incident has caused other injuries, such as fractures to long bones because of falls or high-energy impacts, as in car wrecks. A broken spine can injure the spinal cord to yield a paraplegic, again a difficult challenge for burn workers. The treatment aim becomes survival per se, virtually at any cost to keep the organism alive. There are ethical questions here, of course, such as the utilitarian question how much money should be spent to save a person who will have profound limitations. On a larger scale as has been noted earlier, "cost allocation" (often a euphemism for cutting services) may take the form of closing entire burn units, thus denying or delaying appropriate care for many patients. Such closures result in a form of geographical rationing, since urban centers tend to keep their units open while rural units are lost.

On the other hand, near miraculous techniques can be done to help patients. Surgeons can replace a lost thumb with a big toe, "moving it up." They can build new ears out of rib cartilage, covering them over with the patients' own skin. Modern wheelchairs can give patients surprising mobility, including the ability to drive their own cars. Wigs and cosmetics can do a lot for appearance, for both women and men. A variety of prostheses are available now that are functionally very good and/or visually superb. A missing nose, for example, can be replaced with a prosthesis made from acrylic; by spraying various layers of translucent material, technicians (maybe we should say artists?) create colors and textures that approximate the skin of the patient with remarkable accuracy. A little powder helps cover the edges. Because the colors are so good, because the layers allow the eye to see into the material a bit—as with polished wood—only a trained eye can discern these.

For many of these techniques or devices, the motivation and persistence of the patient is very important: to keep returning to the hospital, to keep putting on make-up, to assure that skin on a stump stays healthy where it rests on an artificial leg. Survivors, especially those in low socio-economic strata and/or with little family support, may not be able to maintain such care.

Some joints become immobile, owing to associated injuries, contractures, long bed-rest, and/or patient unwillingness to work hard in rehab. Heterotopic bone formation, bone growing in a joint and freezing, is extremely difficult to treat: only an entire joint replacement may do the job, and this is expensive and often beyond the psychological range of a patient who has already endured much hospital time. Sometimes the demands on the patient (further operations, rehabilitation, practice at home) seem excessive. He or she may be unwilling, for example, to work at getting further range of motion and strength in an injured hand if the other hand is functioning well. The funds for travel to specialized centers may be unavailable. When the problem is truly intractable, physicians and therapists say, "This is the best we can do with this shoulder; you're going to have to learn to live with it."

This first category of survivors is the smallest, but in many ways the most disturbing to a society which takes perfect health and appearances as a norm. These survivors fly again but on their crippled wings that greatly limit their flights. These are the patients who have narrowly missed death and who, 25 years ago, would surely have died. Social acceptance of their limitations is crucial. What can "normal" people do to welcome them back from their perilous journey?

"Some After-Effects"

This is probably the largest category of survivors, those who leave the unit in pretty good shape, with only a few reminders of the burn and its treatment. We have mentioned many of the common after-effects, and need only to review them here. Their number and persistence give rise to the common phrase "a severe burn lasts forever."

For these patients there has not been heavy structural damage to the body. The actual burn and its damage to skin, then, is the main topic. Most of these patients will be grafted, meaning that they must heal both the graft over the burn as well as the donor site. The donor sites are often maddening because of itching which goes on and on. For some, the itching lasts up to two years. Recent victims love hearing from burn survivors: "Your donor sites will slowly stop itching." Split-thickness skin grafts are so thin that underlying sweat gland, hair follicles, and cushioning fat do not ride along to cover the burn. Grafted sites, therefore, cannot sweat to cool the body. They often feel hot, like a piece of a wool sweater laying over the body. Grafts are thin and easily damaged. Survivors must not expose them to sunburn. The skin may look stretched, shiny, and otherwise irregular, especially if the graft was meshed to yield a pattern of diamond shapes. Grafts may, after some decades, be prone to breaking down or developing cancers, especially in elderly patients. Still more serious problems are contractures over joints, which can be revised by surgery, and hypertrophic scars, very large, hard scars, typically treated by pressure garments. Even flattened scars that look like normal skin tend to restrict movement.

Survivors will usually have general weakness from protracted bedrest, as well as loss of muscle strength, flexibility, and often self-esteem and confidence. These can all be treated, and young patients, in particular, usually rebound very well. Many doctors say, "Make 'em walk early" in order to get patients moving again, both in body and in mind. This is hard to do for a patient covered with bandages and hurting over wide areas of the body, but even a few steps from bed to a chair constitute a victory and a sign that tomorrow may allow for a few further steps. Some physical therapists will put a stop watch on patients, as if for a track event, as they walk down to the water fountain and back. "Great, Mr. Oliver! You did it 30 seconds faster today!" Cheerleaders by nature, physical therapists urge patients on, patients who still feel much doubt and uncertainty: "Will I ever run again?" "Will I ever have sex again?"

"A Good" or Even "Great Result"

This category is the pride and goal of every burn unit. It includes, for example, the perfect graft across the forehead — taken, for example, from the upper arm — with an excellent match for color and texture, so that it cannot be noticed except perhaps when the patient blushes. But even less perfect results are causes for rejoicing. We've seen many patients come back to the units; they are often greeted with cries of, "Oh, it's Mr. Phillips!" or "Mrs. Franklin, how are you?" and "Wow, look at those grafts, they look great" or "Let me see how those ankles turned out!" The patient will often say — even with a smile, "You know, I really hate this place . . . but you guys were great." Seeing such a patient walk, pressure garments and all, is often a high point of the day for burn staff.

Younger patients frequently do very well by virtue of their robust health and their motivation to keep up with their exercises and other aspects of aftercare, not to mention family who will help maintain discipline and support. And, of course, any burns that are less severe in depth and area usually heal better than do larger ones.

These patients fly again and, for the most part, fly very well. For some there are after-effects. Sheffield et al. conclude that "Most patients do well and report a minimal impact of the [burn] illness in their lives and a satisfactory quality of life. A small percentage of the patients (10 percent to 15 percent) have postburn courses complicated by psychiatric problems, noncompliance, and limited ROM [range of motion]" (1988, 176).

Psychological, Social, and Spiritual Aspects

Beyond the state of bones and skin, the patient may re-enter the world with a variety of setbacks and successes. How each patient interprets his or her burn is often a pivotal influence in their recovery beyond the burn unit. Sometimes the ability to resume "activities of daily life" (or ADLs in the physical therapist's abbreviation) depends a lot on mental attitude and the help provided by others.

"Some Grave Difficulties"

As in the most severe physical level above, patients leaving the hospital with considerable psychological difficulties may have had these at the time of the injury. A psychologically disturbed patient who also has burns may go home with all burns healed, but with the mental difficulties — even if treated — no better than before the burn. For other patients, the burn and its sequelae are the cause of psychological difficulty, as in the following case.

Beth Anne was a 24-year-old Wyoming woman severely burned in a car fire. Her extensive wounds were mostly covered by grafts, but her face would need several operations to rebuild her nose. Her surgeon told her that she was doing "very well—right on schedule for this sort of injury," but Beth Anne was intensely angry about her misfortune and current state. "Look at my goddamn photo from before the wreck," she'd snarl, holding up a college photo of her with curled hair, smooth skin, a lovely smile, and pretty eyes. Now only the eyes were the same. "Who the hell will ever want to date me again?"

Lengthy therapy may be able to soften her anger, or it may fail; her grim comment about future dates may be correct, although sometimes it is another survivor who may be attracted to her, meeting her in the unit, during rehab, or in a survivors' group. (We remember a romance of two armless survivors; they would hold hooks.) Beth Anne may have good prospects for a long-term result, but only if she returns for further surgery. Even then, she may be able to see only the disparity between her earlier looks and the final result, and in that disparity see only failure and betrayal.

Some patients lose their sense of the possibility of justice in the world, either as a philosophical or as a religious outlook. "The world is unfair," they may complain, or "No just God would put me through the hell I've been through" or "My God died in that fire."

Families may come apart because of the trauma of a severe burn. Sometimes spouses, unwilling or unable to deal with the burn unit or the demands of aftercare, will divorce the burn victims in their time of greatest need. Naturally, a good burn unit will try to head this off by counseling, home care, and referral to social services or a minister.

"Pretty Much Healed"

This middle range parallels the previous category of physical recovery, patients with some after-effects but a generally good result. The most common psychological problems include anger and depression. If treated, these may fade over time, but for many patients they never completely go away. Some remember the date distinctly, as in "October 12th, when my life changed." Some try to protect themselves on their anniversary date, by being with friends — or by drinking. One woman visits the site of her car fire and leaves flowers. Some refuse to ride in airplanes again or otherwise participate in the source of their burns. (Sometimes it is a spouse who will not let the injured person near such a source.) Some find healing in committing themselves to helping other burn victims by visiting burn units, working in organizations, visiting schools to talk about prevention, and the like.

Some patients find that the burn and its difficult treatment are the source of a new wisdom, a wisdom beyond their chronological years. By reflecting on the severity of their injuries, the injustice of them, and the care of their physicians and nurses, they make new assessments of their own resources and prospects. Young people, especially men in their twenties, sometimes decide to settle down and find a path in life.

We don't mean to overdramatize this, suggesting that all burns are a "crucible of testing that creates wonderful people." Such a formulation is attractive to the unburned, perhaps as a way of assuaging something like survivor's guilt. The underlying assumption might go like this: "I feel so bad that she got burned, but I'll feel better knowing that the time in the hospital changed her life wonderfully forever." We would like the injuring fire to be the biblical refiner's fire, exchanging personal improvement for the burns and suffering. Unfortunately, this is usually not what happens. There are cases of such pivotal changes, but, in our experience, they are rare. They are readily remembered, however, as symbols of something we want to believe. But more commonly survivors have, at best, mixed attitudes about the misfortune of their injury and the good fortune of their healing. At worst, they are depressed and/or angry. (Pruzinski et al. describe some of the psychometric instruments available for assessing patients post-burn; 1992.)

Some patients find a new spiritual outlook that has a deeper sense of absurdity or even evil. A faith that was previously sentimentally optimistic — if it is to survive the burns — eventually must deal with pain, suffering, and injustice. Patients who turn this corner gain spiritual depth and maturity; often, after they are healed, they become very good listeners and counselors for other burn patients.

Some patients find new richness in their relations with family and friends, who are faithful to them during their hospitalization and long recovery at home. One man was deeply touched by the many visits, cards, and other gestures on the part of office-workers and neighbors: "I couldn't believe the outpouring; I had no idea that many people would really care." He believes he healed more quickly, in part because he was motivated to rejoin society.

There has been particular progress in treating burned children, whose re-entry into society is especially difficult. Play therapy has helped both children and adults (Mahaney 1990, Korte et al. 1990). A further extension beyond the hospital is the burn camp; Marion Doctor (1992) describes these and lists 18 of them. The Kids on the Block is a Maryland-based puppet program with over 1,700 community-based groups in the U. S. and other countries; this organization provides puppet shows in schools to help a class prepare to receive a child returning to school post-burn. They also have some 40 other programs addressing medical and educational differences, social concerns, and other disabilities (phone 800-368-KIDS; 301-290-9095 in Maryland).

"More Beautiful Than Before"

We have mentioned this phrase as part of Alan Jeffry Breslau's interpretation of the phoenix, the mythological bird that lives again after perishing in a fire. While the ancient stories describe the bird as the same, Breslau (and others) have found that their post-burn lives are richer and more powerful, in part because they found new resources within themselves as they healed. Another example is the "Guinea Pig Club" from World War II, burned pilots treated in England by Archibald MacIndoe, M.D., who tried various experimental treatments on their dreadful wounds. Those who survived and could do so (and chose to do so) would meet to recall their hard times and to celebrate the survival and victory over their wounds. A film about them (*The Guinea Pig Club*, 1991) has almost a fairy-tale quality, as the survivors speak glowingly, over forty years later, of their treatment and rehabilitation. These reborn Icaruses, flying again, tell a story that is idealized and leaves out the worst features of their original fiery plunge, treatment, and sequelae. Such an outlook may be logical for a person who has suffered much and progressively forgets the worst aspects of the injury and treatment. We do not hear from other guinea pigs who are bitter (or dead) and did not participate in making this upbeat film; for them, the later flights of Icarus are not as high or as wonderful.

How high can a survivor fly? Because there are many levels possible, an easy, single answer would be misleading. We can answer that any flight at all is miraculous from a historical perspective, since virtually all severe burns would have resulted in death 50 years ago. We can answer that death itself, in many religious traditions, is the ultimate and highest kind of flight. We can answer that the stories of burn survivors who "really turn their lives around" are inspiring and comforting to us, whereas we are all too willing to ignore the survivors who have many problems, even including those from before the burn. High-tech burn care can save the lives of burn survivors almost to a miraculous extent, but such survivors will fly at many differing levels, depending on many factors—social, psychological, spiritual, vocational, and more. Ideally, follow-up burn care would deal effectively with all of these, but such an ideal is unlikely to be realized, since we currently invest heavily in emergency and acute care, but not in long-term care.

Chapter Ten
Burn Care as a Stimulus for Medicine and Society

In the first years of the Clinton presidency, the United States was involved in a protracted debate about health care, its structures, financing, and reform. We cannot resolve (or even sketch) the issues here, but we can offer some comments from the burn world that may have implications for health care in America and beyond. By their intense and extreme nature, severe burns have pushed medical thought and practice to insights that are transferable to other areas of medicine and even to society at large. Because burn care itself is not perfect, however, we must first argue for improvements, specifically increased efforts in the two areas of prevention and follow-up after hospitalization.

"The Best Burn" and the Role of Prevention

The best burn is, of course, the burn that never occurs, but America is slow to invest in prevention. Our culture and medical system thrive upon the rescue model: judging by our funding patterns and delivery of medical care, we appear to prefer waiting for emergencies and making the best of them. While we can never prevent all burns, we could prevent many of them if we tried; such efforts would save a lot of money and spare many people much pain. Some prevention strategies are amazingly simple and inexpensive. For example, one common burn among elderly women has been called "the granny gown burn" (Turner and Leman 1989):

> A woman wearing a nightgown cooks over a stove; her long sleeves drag over the burners and ignite. She falls to the ground, her clothes on fire, perhaps sustaining other injuries in the fall.

One solution is simple: large rubber bands worn over the sleeves. Community programs have also stressed not smoking in bed, turning down hot water heaters, and installing smoke alarms. A $10,000 program can prevent several million-dollar burns, certainly a good return on investment.

Some years ago a speaker at a World Burn Congress sponsored by the Phoenix Society (we apologize for not remembering his name) said words to this effect, "I am so tired of posters showing heroic firemen carrying children from fires. The most important point is that such fires should never have happened."

Many fire departments now have programs for schools, community centers, and the like. Some display banners by the firehouse to remind passersby to change the battery in their smoke detectors at Christmas. In the early days of fire detectors a story was repeated in burn circles:

> A fire chief received a fire detector in the mail. Intending to install it but not quite believing in the power of the little gadget, he put it on a shelf on the living room until he could get around to it. One night his house caught on fire. The unit, still in its box, went off, its shrill noise awakening everyone in the house before hot gases could overcome them in their sleep. The next day the fire chief ordered all members of the company to install such detectors in their homes.

There may be some folkloric aspects to this story—including the probable lack of batteries in a boxed unit—but the teaching values are still powerful and illustrative of a revolution in the past ten years. Fire detectors have become widely—but not universally—used. Typically, older homes in poorer sections of a town will have fewer alarms; in such an area a give-away program of smoke alarms can make a large difference. In a project in Oklahoma City, for example, the annualized fire-injury rates declined by 80 percent in the target area during the four years after the distribution of 10,100 smoke alarms (Malonee et al., 1996).

Every Fall the National Fire Protection Association (Quincy, Mass.) sponsors Fire Prevention Week, providing films, brochures, coloring books, and other educational materials for children, families, and adults.

Methodological Problems

Modern burn care knows a lot about the physiology, anatomy, and pharmacology of the human body, but not much about behavior modification and intervention design. How to design and implement prevention programs is poorly understood and research for it is under-funded. Our knowledge of who gets burned and how is limited, since only burn centers currently gather such data, missing all minor burns as well as those treated in other hospitals. New York State requires emergency rooms to report burns over 5 percent TBSA, but this program is designed to detect arsonists, not to evaluate patterns of burn injuries or to create intervention programs. A more focused grant from the New York State Department of Public Health, for example, allows Westchester Country Medical Center to create a project for preventing scalds to toddlers; even here, the methods of chart review may or may not clarify whether such burns are being reduced.

Buildings and Homes

Modern codes that require sprinkler systems, fire-resistant or retardant materials, fire alarms, smoke detectors, fire escapes, marked exits, and the like, effectively reduce risk. Violations of these, however, are common and allow terrible fires that kill many. Recent examples include the Puerto Rico Dupont Plaza Hotel fire of New Year's Eve, 1986, where 96 people died of smoke inhalation, the Bronx Happyland Social Club fire in March of 1990, in which 86 people died, and the 1991 Hamlet, North Carolina, chicken processing plant fire, which killed 25 people. The best codes, if unenforced, will still allow many people to be wounded by burns or to die from them. The large number of illegal sweatshops in New York City virtually predict that another Triangle Shirtwaist disaster will occur. Catastrophes like these gain brief attention in the media but little criminal prosecution follows.

Even small, daily fires are a menace in America: the U.S. ranks first in the western world in deaths and property loss from fire, according to *America Burning* (1973) and its update, *American Burning Revisited* (1988). The first report was sponsored by a national Commission on Fire Prevention and Control and based on two years of hearings and studies. It recommended 90 ways to reduce the risk of fire in buildings and of burn-related injury and death for civilians and firefighters; it called for $125 million a year to implement these recommendations. Annual funding, however, never exceeded $24 million, despite the estimated losses in one year of $11 billion, to say nothing of the thousands of deaths and injuries.

Cigarettes: A Continuing Disaster

According to Sacks and Nelson (1994), fires are the fourth leading cause of death from injury in America, claiming 4,835 lives in 1988 alone. Cigarettes caused an estimated 1,419 of these deaths and 3,766 fire-related injuries; 157 of those who died were children. They conclude: "Smoking is the leading cause of fire death and the second leading cause of fire-related injury in the U. S." (515). They observe that "many residential fires result from a smoldering cigarette igniting bedding or furniture." Other smoking-related injuries stem from children playing with smoking materials, smoking and explosions, cigarettes used in abuse of children, and the role of smoking in car crashes (the driver becomes distracted while handling smoking materials).

Sacks and Nelson also call for a self-extinguishing cigarette. Such a cigarette has been developed but not, unfortunately, produced and marketed. This is tragic, since many burns and deaths could be avoided. Botkin (1988) writes, "While heating equipment and cooking consistently cause the greatest number of residential fires, cigarettes are the single leading cause of residential fire deaths by a wide margin" (226). Most of these are bedding or furniture fires, caused by a smoldering cigarette; the smoker, sleepy and/or intoxicated, typically dies from carbon monoxide poisoning. Improved fabrics, education, and smoke detectors have all contributed to reducing risk, but these are not sufficient. "The most effective potential solution for the cigarette-initiated fire lies with the cigarette itself," Botkin says, but neither governmental force (despite the Cigarette Safety Act of 1984) or industry initiative has brought a self-extinguishing to market. Research has shown that such cigarettes are both technically and commercially feasible. Botkin concludes: "The fire-safe cigarette is an excellent example of preventive medicine that can be pursued through epidemiologic analysis, basic science, effective advocacy, and cooperation between the professions, industry, and government" (229).

Clothing and Fabrics: A Success Story

By 1987, when the Federal Emergency Management Agency did a second evaluation of the nation's fire prevention programs, several positive trends were clear. Fire-related deaths declined, but fire-related injuries remained constant. The most dramatic improvement came in clothing-ignition deaths, thanks to new standards in flammable fabrics, particularly in children's sleepwear.

Contemporary Burn Care

Among the recommendations of the original *America Burning* (1973) was a request of Congress to fund the establishment of 25 burn units and 90 burn programs. No legislative action resulted. Nonetheless, by 1983 there were 125 burn centers in the United States, with one in nearly every major metropolitan area. Two forces behind this growth in specialized care are the Brooke Army Hospital and the Shriners, both already discussed. Worth noting is the link between the two. The Shrine Temples of the Masons, a fraternal organization, has funded hospitals and programs for crippled children since the nineteenth century. With the eradication of polio, it sought a new focus. Curtis Artz, then the commanding officer at Brooke, convinced the Shriners' Past Imperial Potentate, Harvey Beffa, that meeting the needs of burned children would be very rewarding. That year, 1962, the Shriners made a commitment to fund three children's hospitals for burn treatment and research. Like the Brooke Army Hospital, the Shriners Burn Institutes have trained many physicians, who then staff and lead burn units in the U.S. and abroad.

Another source of funding has been firefighters. Although they represent a small percentage of patients in burn centers, their profession is second only to mining in injuries per work hours. Also, they all have personal experience of the devastation that fire can cause. Their support, along with university medical centers, and some — if limited — federal spending, has contributed to the national network of burn centers, burn units, and burn programs we have today.

Burn Statistics

In 1958, when there were fewer than ten hospitals specializing in burn care, the University of Michigan, under the direction of Irving Feller, began to assemble a data base on burns, reviewing 500 burns treated there since 1949. This retrospective study covered mechanism of injury and other severity factors, along with outcome including survival, complications, and deaths. A local burns registry was established for the two Ann Arbor hospitals treating burns, and in 1964 the program expanded to become the National Burn Information Exchange (NBIE), funded by the U. S. Public Health Service. The aims were: to establish standards of care for burn patients; to develop information for improving care by reporting differences in specific techniques, procedures, and practices; to compare methods and results in large numbers of patients; and, finally, to provide information on the etiology of burns that would help create prevention practices (Feller 1987). By 1987, the number of burn units participating had grown from 4 to 50.

The NBIE has learned, for example, that the populations most at risk for fire injuries are the elderly, infants and toddlers, and adult African-American men. More victims come from impoverished circumstances, and these are more often injured at home than at work; they are more likely to live in a multifamily home, lodging, or boarding house than in a private house, and in urban or rural areas rather than the suburbs. Infants and toddlers are more likely to be scalded than burned by flame. The elderly are also at higher risk for scalding. Adolescents are burned often because of high-risk behaviors, typically involving gasoline or home-made incendiaries. Non-elderly adult burns correlate well with smoking and drug or alcohol usage.

Burn statistics help prevention efforts because knowledge of patients helps define populations for education and because understanding of means of injury can lead to changes in products, buildings, and the like. And there are other applications as well: a recent article by Munster, Smith-Meek, and Sharkey demonstrates how computer analysis can show correlations between early surgical intervention, mortality, and cost-effectiveness (1994).

Is Burn Care Perfect?

Modern, high-tech burn care — for all of its strengths and successes — is not perfect. Before extending ideas from the burn world to other areas, therefore, we need to consider some on-going dilemmas in burn care. Indeed, consideration of weaknesses in burn care may help not only burn care itself, but also other areas of medicine.

Coverage, Access, Expense

Some of the most problematic areas of burn care derive from its emergency nature. Burn care works very well for a small number of patients who are evenly spaced throughout any given year. A large burn disaster, however, will immediately overload the two or three closest units. Air ambulances can further distribute patients, but only at large expense and inconvenience to family and friends. The picture is even more difficult if we consider international aspects. The large number of excellent burn units in the United States are routinely not accessible to citizens of Mexico, the Caribbean, or Latin America. Even rural patients in the United States may not have ready access — and anyone may be denied access unintentionally because family or even physicians underestimated the severity of the burn injury. Such patients may get to the unit days late and with infected wounds. Discharged patients often have financial problems that make return visits to centers impossible, especially if insurance coverage is lacking or the distance is considerable.

Finally, the highest technologies in burn care simply are not available world-wide, especially in poorer countries. It is easy for Americans to think that modern burn technology will change burn care everywhere, but for every patient receiving superb care in the United States and Europe, there are scores of patients in other countries receiving care at a pre-1950 level. Some, of course, receive no care at all because of problems of geographical access, lack of sufficient burn units, even religious beliefs and folk-medicine practices that do not include hospital care. For them, burn care pre-dates the twentieth century, and will usually lead to scars, contractures, infections, and death. There is a further, complex issue: is high-tech, high-expense treatment the best way to go? Some lower cost treatments, in Brazil for example, get equally good results when measured by survival after hospitalization.

Follow-Up for Patients

Perhaps the weakest stage in modern burn care is follow-up after the hospital stay, as previously discussed. This is a great pity, since all the other stages have been typically very good. Emergency care in the U. S. is the best in the world, although it has the limits just described (high numbers, as in disasters, and service to rural areas). Burn unit technology and protocols are typically superb, including the contributing professionals who begin rehabilitation. But once the patient is "out the door," continuity of care falls off dramatically. Yes, there are clinic dates which many patients keep, but social problems for patients re-entering ordinary life are often difficult, and our current system pays little attention to patients after their hospital course. This is an area for improvement in burn care as well as in other fields of medicine — not to mention the society at large, which routinely shortchanges sick and disabled persons of all ages, but especially the young, the elderly, and the poor, both urban and rural.

Finances

Again, this is a complex subject not to be adequately covered here, but our system of high-tech burn care can only work with a small number of patients and a constant flow of dollars from insurers, donors, the sponsoring hospital, fraternal groups, or other sources. Total expenses for a burn patient may easily total $500,000, and a million-dollar burn is not uncommon. If needs increase in America, the burn units as now organized will not be able to handle the load. Some hospitals have been closing their burn units — famous as money losers — further exacerbating the dilemma. One of the most effective uses of burn-care dollars is, of course, prevention, discussed below. A $10,000 program in safety awareness may prevent a single $1,000,000 burn — a 100 percent return on dollars invested.

Hierarchies and Medical Politics

Burn units typically try to promote a democratic set of values among the caregivers, whether techs, nurses, or surgeons. Many of them have made great progress, while some, regrettably, are still fairly hierarchical. Probably all units could benefit from further efforts to reduce all kinds of hierarchy and prejudice, including racism, sexism, and homophobia. Hospital politics — always complex — are often an obstacle for burn care, which is expensive, labor-intensive, and space-demanding; other hospital services often try to scavenge resources from burn units, requiring time and savvy from the medical director to fend them off. Fostering better relations between all hospital services should be an aim of hospital administration and burn units as well. Some burn physicians serve as consultants for other services, using their extensive experience with infections, moribund patients, multisystem failure, and the like; such collaboration keeps them from being isolated in their highly specialized world and allows a cross-fertilization among intelligent and sympathetic minds.

The improvements in burn care discussed above would serve patients, their families, and staff; these ideals may well help improve other areas of medicine as well. Turning now to areas where burn care has excelled, we can speculate about implications for the hospital and beyond.

Strengths of Modern Burn Care

We have already described many features of modern burn care that take medical thinking, technology, and patient care to advanced levels. Burn care brings together various resources in ways that may be useful and inspiring to other areas of medicine.

Whole Person Approach

The very nature of burns and their sequelae have caused burn care-givers to consider the patient as a totality of systems: skin, lungs, circulation, psychology, as we saw in Chapter 3. When burn care is best practiced, the patient is viewed as a whole, every part connecting to every other; as care of different aspects of the patient intersect, there are synergistic benefits. For example, care of diet, wounds, and the patient's psychological needs will probably influence his or her immune strength. Concern for family and other visitors will help the patient in the short and the long runs. Attention to the patient's life beyond the hospital — vocational, recreational, and attitudinal — will increase his or her motivation to protect the grafts, keep follow-up appointments, and the like.

This whole-person approach has extended to other areas of medicine; family practice, for example, has been a leader. But some specialties still focus so closely on organ systems, behaviors, or cells, that the emotional needs of the patient are lost; critics have argued that such an approach can compromise patient satisfaction and even healing to the extent that lawsuits are more likely. Furthermore, patients with intractable conditions are more likely to try bizarre (and often expensive and/or harmful) alternatives to medicine if their emotional and spiritual needs are not met.

Interdisciplinary Staffing and Team Approach

Reflecting the various needs of the patient are the various medical disciplines that make up the burn team approach: physicians, nurses, occupational therapists, physical therapists, dietitians, and often specialists from such areas as pulmonary care, psychology, psychiatry, pastoral care, social work, and speech therapy. The burn unit is arguably the most interdisciplinary service in the hospital, and the burn profession has made the notion of the "burn team" a central concept. The burn team includes all the disciplines just mentioned and suggests that, like an athletic team, all these varied roles are important to the common goal of healing the patient.

There are some implications for this. First, there is (ideally) an atmosphere of mutual respect in which everyone realizes that all disciplines have their standards, professionalism, and specific contributions to make to the patient. These attitudes are important motivators for burn care workers, who, as we have seen, sometimes find the continuous stress of the unit so overwhelming that they transfer to easier services. "One of the things that keeps me going up here — besides seeing the patients get better," one nurse said, "is that everyone takes what I do seriously." It is hard to overestimate that power of professional validation by others; such positive feedback is a reward and a source of encouragement beyond what salary can provide. Sutton (1993) emphasizes the need to help caregivers in their first 12 months in the unit, a time of particularly high stress.

The standard daily or weekly rounds become a ritual in recognizing the cooperating strengths of the various disciplines. Each discipline sends a representative, often a senior or administrative member, to the meeting; each person has the right — and duty — to speak, to listen, and to answer questions. The person who leads the meeting (typically, a physician) may ask for information about a particular patient from, say, the dietitian, the social worker, the occupational therapist, or the psychiatrist. In rounds we've observed or participated in, the physician sets a standard of mutual respect by speaking to the various specialties with equal interest, importance, and deference. At St. Luke's Regional Medical Center, Sioux City, Iowa, the Burn Trauma Unit has extended the team concept to a shared governance model, which gives nurses more decision-making power than in a centralized structure. The team concept also permeates the American Burn Association. This group, founded in 1967, meets yearly, with representatives from all disciplines involved. There is, however, room for improvement in the democratization of this organization: all presidents through 1995 have been medical doctors; further, all have been men.

Some burn units consider the patients themselves as members of the team, not as primary care-givers, of course, but as the focus for healing and the future bearer of responsibility: for taking meds, wearing pressure garments, attending therapy sessions, coming to clinic follow-up, and the like. "But Mr. Turley, you are the star of this team!" one nurse repeatedly exhorted a gloomy patient, until he accepted and even enjoyed the idea. Another variation in the burn team concept involves regional coverage when no burn unit is centrally located. Thus the "burn team" in the Billings, Montana region has served the relatively small population of 330,000 over the large area of 50,000 square miles. This consortium provides rotating services by physicians and registered nurses. Some patients remain within their region while healing; others are referred to the nearest burn unit 650 miles away (Peet et al. 1993).

Every clinic or service in a hospital can benefit from the team concept and from the validation that should accompany it. Such support is especially important to workers who are lower on the pay scale, and it helps improve morale for everyone. This makes possible more loving and attentive care to patients and their families — not to mention a decrease in errors.

Family and Friends

Well run burn units pay particular attention to patients' family members, who are potentially the prime motivators for the patients. But families usually know nothing about burn units and find much in them that is frightening. Staff should do their best to educate families about the sights and sounds of the unit, the ups and downs of burn patients, and the general course of treatment, especially the landmarks of improvement. Family members, however well educated, cannot immediately hear everything that is said in the emotionally charged unit; they need repeated information, well beyond the redundancy considered normal. Some units make publications available for family to take home; others may have a VCR in the waiting room with videotapes explaining aspects of the burn unit. Extra copies should be available to loan for home viewing.

As discharge time comes closer, a social worker or nurse will study the patient's prospects for care beyond the unit. Since initially most patients cannot drive, are drivers available for clinic visits? Can this child, flown in by helicopter, get physical therapy at a local hospital? Are Medicare and Medicaid available to this patient? What about home health care? Such effort to view a patient in the context of a supportive social network is a concept that can benefit every area of medicine.

Other Social Networks

Some burn units (some 58 percent, according Mapp et al. 1993) sponsor burn survivor support groups. These usually have monthly meetings, although sometimes weekly; topics include functional, cosmetic, and social problems, as well as dealing with pain, returning to work, and resolving drug problems.

Some burn units refer patients to local support groups. The largest of these is the Phoenix Society for Burn Survivors (11 Rust Hill Road, Levittown, PA 19056-2311). This organization has over 300 chapters in the U. S. and 65 in other countries. It sponsors several burn camps as well as an annual World Burn Congress. Its newsletter *The Icarus File* includes articles on burn survivors, news of treatment and prevention, and lists of appropriate books and home-care products.

Another support group is the National Burn Victims Foundation (P. O. Box 409, 246 Myersville Rd., Basking Ridge, NJ 07920). This group has disaster response teams (with some 1,000 volunteers) for burns and other accidents. It also works in several areas, including child abuse, counselling for fire-setters, mental-health and forensics.

The Burns United Support Group (P. O. Box 36416, Grosse Pointe Farms, MI 48236) serves Michigan area survivors through three chapters. This organization helps children and adults, regardless of the size of the burn, and emphasizes emotional care of family and friends. Support groups are peer-led.

The Lightning Strike and Electric Shock Victims International group (214 Canterbury Rd., Jacksonville, NC 28450) holds annual meetings, offers support in establishing groups, and emphasizes long-term effects for survivors.

Children recovering from burns are cared for at several camps especially designed for them (Doctor, cited in Chapter 9). Such children feel strange with "normal" children but get along well with wounded peers, comparing burns, length of hospital stay, and the like, much like baseball statistics.

The Rancho Los Amigos Hospital in Downey, California, has an Image Enhancement Center to help patients (regardless of the source of their injury) deal with their new body configurations, abilities, and appearances. At Tampa General Hospital, Chaplain Robert G. Wiley directs a program of two-day trauma/burn seminars for clergy. Over four years some 36 care-givers were trained (Wiley 1993).

Many other injuries, diseases, and syndromes have similar support groups. *The Self-Help Source Book* (White and Madara 1995) lists and describes hundreds of groups in the areas of abuse, addictions, bereavement, disabilities, health (both physical and mental), and so on. Such groups can be extremely helpful; care-givers should refer patients to them and work with them so the groups have the most recent and accurate information. (For a discussion of bioethical aspects of the self-help revolution, see Carter 1995.)

The whole person approach, interdisciplinary staffing and team concept, the consideration of the roles of family and friends, the use of support networks—many of these concepts from the burn world have been used elsewhere in medicine. We salute such use and call for even further applications for the following reasons: patients respond better; there is less stress on family and friends; and medical personnel benefit from having cooperation from several sources.

Epilogue

In this book we have attempted to show the complexity of the world of burns and the many sorts of responses humans have made to fire and burns. Meanings and treatments have varied widely for many reasons — historical, social, cultural — and, of course, according to the various points of view: those of patients, family members, caregivers, and outsiders to the burn world. Meanings and treatments have influenced each other as well. A given definition of a wound will influence how it is treated, whether by first-aiders or by professionals. Treatments have evolved over time, especially in the past generation, changing the meanings of burns. Survival of patients with severe burns is now all but miraculous compared to earlier treatments, and the results — through grafting, therapy, rehabilitation, and psychiatric care — are well beyond mere survival.

In these closing pages, we would like (1) to summarize some recommendations and (2) to pay tribute to the many persons who have grappled with severe burns one way or another, bringing their resources to confront this formidable wound.

Recommendations

We call for increased efforts, money, and cooperation in the area of prevention; we need safer cars, homes, and workplaces. Tobacco in all forms should continue to disappear. We call for less use of alcohol and illegal drugs and for the healing of social conditions that invite their abuse.

We call for better ways of following-up patients: home-care, transportation, discharge planning, and communication between hospitals and patients following discharge.

We call for policies from the government (Social Security, Medicare, Medicaid, etc.) and the insurance industry that support both prevention and rehabilitation.

We call for a wider network of burn-care facilities and for treatments that are less expensive than the state-of-the-art, high-tech treatments that now typify burn units.

We call for greater sensitivity toward persons who have survived burns and other trauma and other serious illness such as AIDS; may we listen to them well and offer our support.

We call for positive images of survivors of burns and other trauma in fiction, film, and other popular arts. Artistic treatments nourish the social imagination; these are as necessary to a society as medical treatments because they help us understand a wholeness that can embrace fear, pain, and despair.

Tributes to People in the World of Burns

First, naturally, we pay tribute to persons who have survived severe burns. They are all different in their backgrounds and in their outcomes from their burns, but they have in common the experience of devastating injury and long recovery. They are as different as Eva Le Gallienne, the actress who survived a propane explosion and subsequent disfigurement in the first half of the twentieth century (Schanke 1992) and Dax Cowart, who survived a similar explosion (while losing fingers and eyesight) to become a personal injury attorney (*Icarus File* 1996).

We pay tribute to burn-care workers: nurses, physicians, therapists, techs, unit clerks, nutritionists, counsellors, psychiatrists, social workers, chaplains, and many more; all these have dealt with distressing wounds and difficult mental states of their patients, with little reward, acknowledgment, and certainly no public fame. Many survivors, however, have learned first-hand of the care and expertise of these workers, and some have expressed their thanks in words, letters, or even plaques. One plaque, on display at the Tampa Bay Regional Burn Unit, has been carefully crafted at home. It is constructed in the shape of a heart, about the size of two open hands, cut from wood. The message is typed on ordinary typing paper, and the paper has been singed black along the edges then sealed in clear acrylic. The text reads:

A special touch, A kind thought, A caring disposition . . . these are characteristics of the very special people who work the burn unit at Tampa General. There aren't enough words to express our sincere thanks for the very special care that I received during my stay . . . the many kind deeds, the friendship, companionship, and moral support that helped guide me along the road to recovery. Please accept this plaque as a symbol of our heartfelt gratitude.

— Skip Dyke & Family

We have seen similar plaques in other units; sometimes there is a photo of a child, scarred but smiling. Sometimes the plaque is from local firefighters, who are perennial donors to burn units.

Finally, we wish to acknowledge the heroism of persons who have confronted burns in various other ways: we think of family members, co-workers, neighbors, and others who have rallied around a burn patient. We think also of artists and thinkers who have explored the nature of extremity, who have celebrated the efforts of others to meet and confront desperate situations, and who have attempted to express the inexpressible, grappling with the limits of images and words, imagination, mind, and spirit.

At the end of *The Plague*, Albert Camus presents his narrator, Dr. Rieux, observing the celebration of the town of Oran, where the plague is finally over, where fireworks — harming no one — now shoot into the night sky. The passage well illustrates some of the urges that prompted this book:

And it was in the midst of shouts rolling against the terrace wall in massive waves that waxed in volume and duration, while cataracts of colored fire fell thicker through the darkness, that Dr. Rieux resolved to compile this chronicle, so that he should not be one of those who hold their peace but should bear witness in favor of those plague-stricken people; so that some memorial of the injustice and outrage done them might endure; and to state quite simply what we learn in time of pestilence; that there are more things to admire in men then to despise.

Nonetheless, he knew that the tale he had to tell could not be one of final victory. It could be only the record of what had had to be done, and what assuredly would have to be done again in the never ending fight against terror and its relentless onslaughts, despite their personal afflictions, by all who, while unable to be saints but refusing to bow down to pestilences, strive their utmost to be healers. (Camus, 286–87)

For us, this passage describes the people and events of the burn world, interprets the difficulty and complexity of this world, and salutes all those who pass through it, as patient, as burn-worker, as family or friend.

Camus ends his novel with the reminder that such threats as plagues are always with us "for the bane and enlightenment" of persons. Burns, as well, will always be with us. May we learn from them, support those who deal with them, and comfort those who suffer them.

Appendix 1: Versions of the Phantom

This appendix presents a brief overview of the many versions of the Phantom made into film in the past fifty years. They demonstrate the continuing fascination and economic value the character has had in contemporary popular culture. Within the genre we notice the wide range of themes films take from previous versions, some ingenious variations, others pallid exploitations. Nearly all are readily available on video, indicating their continuing impact on our imagining of the burn patient/victim/monster.

1941. *The Face Behind the Mask*, written specifically for Peter Lorre. In this version, Lorre plays a Hungarian watchmaker whose face is burned in a tenement fire. Impoverished, wearing a blank mask, and rejected by potential employers, Lorre contemplates suicide before turning to crime. He is "saved" when he meets a sympathetic young blind girl. The romance doesn't last long, however, for she is killed by gangsters just before the marriage, and Lorre sets out on revenge, resuming his evil career.

1941. *A Woman's Face* with Joan Crawford. In this version an ugly woman is rejected by society but made beautiful by plastic surgery. She returns to break the hearts of the men who had rejected her. Ugliness on the outside, it appears, has created evil on the inside, which a new, superficial beauty cannot reverse. Thus it is society's fault for valuing beauty over character and for making ugly people suffer in such a way that others suffer as well.

1943. *Phantom of the Opera*. This version, like the silent version, was also produced by Universal studios. It was filmed in Technicolor, and redesigned as a musical starring Nelson Eddy as the dashing Lieutenant and Claude Rains as the Phantom. The young singer, Christine, was played by Susanna Foster, intended by the studio to replace Jeannette MacDonald, Eddy's long-standing singing partner. The film is a luxurious production despite its production during World War II. The restructuring of the story line into a musical with comedic intention diminishes the evil nature of the Phantom, making him more pathetic than frightening. The original set of the silent version was used in the filming, but little of the original story remains. The Phantom's makeup, intended to represent an acid burn of the face, lacks any resemblance to real disfigurement. The film, though deficient by our (the authors') standard, was a box office hit. This success may have contributed to subsequent interest in re-filming the story.

1944. *The Climax*. This film, starring Boris Karloff was conceived as a sequel to the '43 version of the Phantom, using the same opera house set on Stage 28 (this set still exists and is part of the Universal Studios tour). The story line included the reincarnation of a murdered diva, played by Susanna Foster. Without explaining how he has survived the previous film ending, the Phantom has returned and believes that the character played by Foster is the soprano murdered in the previous version by the spectacular falling chandelier. This film was neither a commercial or a critical success.

1953. *House of Wax*. Considered one of the best 3-D films ever produced, this Vincent Price vehicle portrays a mad sculptor, who with his cape, wide brimmed hat, and severe facial disfigurement clearly evokes the original Lon Chaney *Phantom*. It was this role that made Price a horror film star.

1954. *The Queen of Outer Space*. In this cult classic (with a minor role played by Nancy Davis, a.k.a. Reagan), Zsa Zsa Gabor stars as an evil masked figure, the queen of an all-female planet, Venus. Her burned face (radiation this time) is exposed by a team of American astronauts who defeat and kill her. The make-up showing her disfigurement is better than Claude Rain's. Although this film is not an obvious version of the *Phantom*, the dramatic sequence of manipulation, discovery, rescue of the beautiful maiden, and necessary death of the masked evil queen (perhaps a genius) qualify it for inclusion.

1956. *Fire Maidens of Outer Space*. This film, only slightly less memorable than *Queen of Outer Space*, is known for its lavish poster depicting the burned and blackened Fire Maiden embracing the traditional damsel in distress "dedicated to the purpose of creating a race of supermen." It is one of a large number of films made cheaply in the 1950s that combined themes of outer space exploration and lost colonies of lonely women — typically described as Amazons — who are "rescued" by brave spac*emen*. Fire, flames, or radiation injuries of some type are nearly always included as part of the plot. And those who are so disfigured are doomed to die. The sexual imagery, a continuing dynamic tension in all the *Phantoms*, is exaggerated to absurd lengths in this and related pieces of the period.

1955. *El Fantasma de la Opereta*. This South American film, produced by the Argentinean film-maker Carrerra, is the first "black-comedy" version of the Phantom.

1957. *Man of a Thousand Faces*. James Cagney plays the Phantom among other roles in this biography of Lon Chaney. The film accurately portrays the terrific efforts Chaney put into creating his roles, including the kind of pain required to contort his body and use the make-up that he designed himself. As the Phantom, for example, he inserted wires into his nose to get the flared and upturned nostrils characteristic of severely burned faces, used drugged eye drops to achieve his bug-eyed appearance, and placed disks inside his cheeks to create the flat expressionless demeanor that made the face so horrifying when the Phantom is first unmasked (see Figure 14).

1960. *Eyes Without a Face (Les yeux sans visage)*. Although the facial disfigurement in this Georges Franju classic is the result of an auto accident, the smooth porcelain mask worn by the mad surgeon's daughter is the traditional Phantom cover-up. Shot in black and white, the story of the father's attempt to restore his daughter's face by stealing the faces of other young girls creates a haunting and horrifying movie. The climax, when she realizes what her father is doing, and the dungeon-like morgue of their home-research lab, recall the opera underground scenes of the original silent *Phantom* of 1925.

1960. *Phantasma de la Opereta*. Directed by Fernando Cortes, this starred the comedian Tin-Tan described by Perry (1987) as an inexpensive parody comedy version that has been lost and was not viewed by the author (JAP).

1962. *Phantom of the Opera*. Herbert Lom stars in this Roger Corman rendition. This was the first full-scale, expensive Hammer production intended to be a major first-run release, but it bombed at the box office. This Phantom did not live up to Hammer horror expectations despite the gratuitous inclusion of eye stabbing and hangings. The plot proceeds as a love story with a disfigured servant, a dwarf, who provides the chief horror element as he serves his master, the Phantom. The location for the film, the Wimbledon Theater in London, became the stage for a theatrical production of the Phantom in 1975.

1971. *The Abominable Dr. Phibes*. This film is described in the *Encyclopedia of Horror Movies* as a cross between the psycho-killer plot and *The Phantom of the Opera*. It stars Vincent Price in his 100th film role. *Variety* called it "an anachronistic period horror musical camp fantasy." An additional plot twist had Dr. Phibes recreating the biblical plagues of Egypt against the doctors he held responsible for his own fate and the death of his wife. A sequel the following year, *Dr. Phibes Rises Again*, continued the revenge of the facially maimed doctor.

1974. *The Phantom of Hollywood*. This made-for-TV movie transforms the opera house into a film studio. Its main purpose seems to have been to capitalize on the dramatic possibilities of studio renovations. The destruction of large blocks of old sets was incorporated into the filming.

1974. *Phantom of the Paradise*. This rock opera is the first film by Brian DePalma. The story combines elements of previous *Phantom* versions and *Faust*. The mask used by this Phantom is like the head of a bird. The Phantom is a composer, burned in a fire at a record factory owned by an "unscrupulous impresario" (played by the composer Paul Williams), who has made a pact with the devil. The film combines themes from Faust and the *Phantom*, images of the Phoenix (both the bird-like mask and the name of the female singer), and sub-plots of murder to create a confusing and ineffective mix. But it is fun to watch and contains intimations of the creative horror film abilities of DePalma that appear in his later films.

1982. *Phantom of the Opera* (CBS). This version was also made for television and is set in Hungary before World War I. This Phantom is first set aflame and then doused with acid. The plot line is not linear, relying on time jumps to build a story of two young heroines played by the same actress, appearing first as the pre-burned Phantom's first wife and then as his post-injury ingenue. This and other devices are distracting and unnecessary, making the film dramatically unsatisfying.

1989. *Phantom of the Opera.* Starring Robert Englund, it capitalizes on England's fame as Freddy Krueger in *Nightmare on Elm Street.* It is an awful film.

This film listing is not complete but represents accessible versions of the type. *Darkman II* and *III*, endless *Nightmares on Elm Street,* and other burned face movies are not included in order to emphasize the most directly related images only.

Appendix 2: A Room Fire Illustrates Modern Fire Science

Fire is a form of rapid oxidation, dependent on the factors that initiate and sustain it: a combustible fuel, an oxidizer (usually oxygen in gas form) available in sufficient quantity, and energy for ignition. When fire burns, it does so at such a rate that the chemical reactions involved generate heat and light. (Rust, another form of oxidation, is so slow that the energy released is imperceptible.) Fire is divided into two kinds: (1) *glowing*, in which there is fire with an absence of flame, such as charcoal; and (2) *flaming*, in which there is a combustion of superheated gases. These occur as the incandescent flames we typically think of as the flames of fire, but also as explosions, or nearly instantaneous flames — such as the "flash-over" much feared by fire-fighters — that are beyond human perception. The energy released by the chain reaction in a self-sustaining fire is expressed as heat and light. The degree of heat released depends on the rate of reaction. Heat and light are dissipated from a fire at a rate dependent on the surrounding environment. Our discussion derives from the standard textbooks of fire science including Bare (1978) and Roblee, McKechnie, and Lundy (1981).

Heat is transferred during the fire by several means, all of which can cause further ignition. *Conduction* is the transmission of heat through a substance with no visible motion or alteration in the substance; this is the principle used in an electric stove. *Convection* is the transmission of heat through the motion of that substance. As air passes over a heated metal, such as a wall heater, it rises. In a fire, it is this energy transfer which moves smoke upward. Convection works equally well with gases and liquids. *Radiation* is the transfer of heat energy in a straight line from the source, such as the rays of the sun. Although we generally consider a fire to spread by direct contact, all three methods are important factors in the spread of fires. The sequence of events in a typical room fire illustrates these principles. Fire science divides the progress of a fire into several stages:

Incipient. At the beginning of a room fire, there is an open flame, a glowing fire, or some other heat source, in the presence of normal oxygen levels

(21 percent of normal air) at ordinary room temperature (50–80° F), and an appropriate fuel (fabric, paper, wood). Convection to the heat source draws oxygen in. At this stage no fire or smoke may be visible.

Smoldering. As heat intensity increases, convection and conduction raise the heat level of the fuel source to the ignition point of the fuel. Little flame is visible at this stage, but smoke is obvious.

Flame. The fire in this early stage has a high content of the products of combustion, because the heat level is relatively low and the oxygen supply is being used up; the smoke is thick and heavy. As heat and smoke rise, however, fresh oxygen is drawn into the base of the fire. If the heat is high enough and oxygen readily available, the mass of flammable gases reach a critical level and a flash point with full flame, relatively clear smoke, and high heat takes over the room. This moment, also known as "flash-over," can be fast and violent. Anyone present would be killed immediately.

Heat. At this stage fire spreads by direct contact and radiant heat, which can ignite objects remote from the flame source. In a room fire, heat is the most important factor in the fire's spread, operating through conduction, convection, and radiation.

The duration of each of these stages depends on many factors: fuel availability and its arrangement (the structure of a bonfire is important to starting and maintaining the fire), humidity, the availability of oxygen, wind (or, in the case of a house fire, open doors and windows), and other factors.

We can illustrate these elements more specifically. Let's say a man has fallen asleep on a sofa and that he has dropped a cigarette between its cushions, where it smolders. Even this stage of the fire might be enough to kill him as oxygen levels fall and carbon monoxide levels rise. The presence of a smoke detector would provide early warning of the smoke, before unconsciousness occurred. The smoldering might not progress to flame unless a door or window were opened, causing a backdraft. If enough oxygen is available the entire room would become engulfed in flame, unless the contents and construction material were especially flame-resistant or flame-retardant.

Fighting such a fire employs the same principles: the fire needs heat, oxygen, and fuel to maintain combustion. Firefighters pour water into the living room reducing heat, cooling potential fuels, and maybe even shutting off oxygen flow by covering the fuel. Removing nearby fuel (such as dragging out smoldering furniture) will further limit a fire's growth.

Bibliography/Filmography

Introduction

Arturson, C. 1992. "Analysis of Severe Fire Disasters." In *Management of Mass Burn Casualties and Fire Disasters*, ed. M. Marsellis and S. W. A. Gunn. Dordrecht: Kluwer.
Osler, William. 1904. *Aequanimitas with Other Addresses*. Philadelphia: P. Blakiston's Son and Co.

Chapter 1

Blakiston's Gould Medical Dictionary. 1979. 4th ed. New York: McGraw-Hill.
Blumenfield, Michael and Margot M. Schoeps. 1993. *Psychological Care of the Burn and Trauma Patient.* Baltimore: Williams and Wilkins.
Breslau, Alan Jeffry. 1977. *The Time of My Death: A Story of Miraculous Survival.* New York: E. P. Dutton.
Bringgold, Diane. 1979. *Life Instead.* Ventura, Calif.: Howard Publishing.
Brown, Larry. 1994. *On Fire.* Chapel Hill, N.C.: Algonquin.
Carter, Albert Howard, III. 1989. "Metaphors in the Physician-Patient Relationship." *Soundings* 72, 1 (Spring): 153–64.
Coover, Robert. 1977. *The Public Burning.* New York: Viking.
Crane, Stephen. 1899. "The Monster." *Great Short Works.* New York: Harper and Row, 1968.
Darkman. 1990. (film) . Universal City Studios.
Dorland's Illustrated Medical Dictionary. 1988. 27th ed. Philadelphia: W. B. Saunders.
Ehrlich, Gretel. 1994. *A Match to the Heart.* New York: Pantheon.
Forbes, Esther. 1943. *Johnny Tremain, a Novel for Old and Young.* New York: Dell. 1961.
Goffman, Erving. 1963. *Stigma: Notes on the Management of Spoiled Identity.* New York: Simon and Schuster, 1986.
Grealy, Lucy. 1993. "Mirrorings: To Gaze upon My Reconstructed Face." *Harper's* (February): 66–75.
———. 1994. *Autobiography of a Face.* New York: Houghton Mifflin.
Harkins, Henry N. 1942. *The Treatment of Burns.* Springfield, Ill.: Charles C. Thomas.
Maher, Ellen L. 1989. "Burnout: Metaphors of Destruction and Purgation." *Soundings* 72, 1 (Spring): 27–37.
March, Joseph Moncure. 1994. *The Wild Party: The Lost Classic.* Illus. Art Spiegelman. New York: Pantheon.
May, William F. 1991. *The Patient's Ordeal.* Bloomington: Indiana University Press.

Munster, Andrew M. et al. 1993. *Severe Burns: A Family Guide to Medical and Emotional Recovery*. Baltimore: Johns Hopkins University Press.

Ondaatje, Michael. 1993. *The English Patient*. New York: Vintage.

Petro, Jane A. and C. Andrew Salzberg. 1992. "Ethical Issues of Burn Management." *Clinics in Plastic Surgery* 19, 3 (July): 615–21.

Please Let Me Die. Videotape Library of Psychiatric Disorders, vol. 129, May 1974.

Rothenberg, Maria and Mel White. 1985. *David*. New York: Berkley.

Sacks, Oliver. 1984. *A Leg to Stand On*. New York: Harper and Row.

Scarry, Elaine. 1985. *The Body in Pain: The Making and Unmaking of the World*. New York: Oxford University Press.

Shelley, Mary. 1818. *Frankenstein*. New York: Collier, 1961.

Shulman, Alix Kates. 1974. *Burning Questions*. New York: Knopf.

Snitker, David. 1983. *I Can Make It One More Day*. Newell, Iowa: Bireline Pub. Co.

Stedman's Medical Dictionary. 1990. 25th ed. Baltimore: Williams and Wilkins.

Ton, Mary Ellen. 1982. *The Flames Shall Not Consume You*. Elgin, Ill.: David C. Cook.

Wolfe, Tom. 1979. *The Right Stuff*. New York: Farrar, Straus and Giroux.

Chapter 2

Ansari, Saeed M. 1992. "Domestic Fire Problems in Third World Countries." In *The Management of Mass Burn Casualties and Fire Disasters*, ed. M. Masellis and S. W. A. Gunn. Dordrecht: Kluwer, 1992.

Bedier, Joseph, ed. 1945. *The Romance of Tristan and Iseult*. Trans. Hilaire Belloc. New York: Random House.

Blumenfield, Michael and Margot M. Schoeps. 1993. *Psychological Care of the Burn and Trauma Patient*. Baltimore: Williams and Wilkins.

Esslin, Martin. 1969. *Theater of the Absurd*. New York: Doubleday.

Gone with the Wind. 1939. (film). MGM.

International Dictionary of Medicine and Biology. 1986. 3 vols. New York: John Wiley and Sons.

Maclean, Norman. 1992. *Young Men and Fire*. Chicago: University of Chicago Press.

Munster, Andrew M. 1994. "Burns in India." *Journal of Burn Care and Rehabilitation* 15, 3: 260–68.

The New Larousse Encyclopedia of Mythology. 1968. Trans. Richard Aldington and De-Lano Ames. Middlesex: Hamlyn.

Ovid. *Metamorphoses*. 1955. Trans. Rolfe Humphries. Bloomington: Indiana University Press.

Renz, Barry M. and Roger Sherman. 1992. "Automobile Carburetor- and Radiator-Related Burns." *Journal of Burn Care and Rehabilitation* 13, 4 (July/August): 414–21.

St. Petersburg Times. 1990. "Parasailer Rescued from Power Lines." 28 June, 4B, col. 1.

Chapter 3

Blumenfield, Michael and Patricia M. Reddish. 1987. "Identification of Psychologic Impairment in Patients with Mild-Moderate Thermal Injury: Small Burn, Big Problem." *General Hospital Psychiatry* 9: 142–46.

Blumenfield, Michael and Margot M. Schoeps. 1993. *Psychological Care of the Burn and Trauma Patient*. Baltimore: Williams and Wilkins.

Budny, P. G., P. J. Regan, and A. H. N. Roberts. 1991. "Ritual Burns: The Buddhist Tradition." *Burns* 17: 335–37.

Keneally, Thomas. *1994. Schindler's List.* New York: Simon and Schuster.

Kushner, Harold S. 1981. *When Bad Things Happen to Good People.* New York: Avon.

Lifton, Robert J. 1986. *The Nazi Doctors: Medical Killing and the Psychology of Genocide.* New York: Basic Books.

MacLeish, Archibald. 1958. *J.B.* Boston: Houghton Mifflin.

Rothenberg, Maria and Mel White. 1985. *David.* New York: Berkley.

Schindler's List. 1993. (film). Universal.

Soelle, Dorothee. 1984. *Suffering.* Trans. Everett R. Kalin. Philadelphia: Fortress Press.

Vonnegut, Kurt, Jr. 1969. *Slaughterhouse Five.* New York: Dell.

Whose Life Is It Anyway? 1981. (film). MGM.

Chapter 4

Blumenfeld, Michael and Patricia M. Reddish. 1987. "Identification of Psychologic Impairment in Patients with Mild-Moderate Thermal Injury: Small Burn, Big Problem." *General Hospital Psychiatry* 9: 142–46.

Clark, Brian. 1978. *Whose Life Is It Anyway?* New York: Dell.

Imbus, Sharon and Bruce Zawacki. 1977. "Autonomy for Burned Patients When Survival Is Unprecedented." *New England Journal of Medicine* 297: 308.

——. 1986. "Encouraging Dialogue and Autonomy in the Burn Intensive Care Unit." *Critical Care Clinics* 2, 1: 53–60.

Kliever, Lonnie D., ed. 1989. *Dax's Case: Essays in Medical Ethics and Human Meaning.* Dallas: Southern Methodist University Press.

May, William F. 1991. *The Patient's Ordeal.* Bloomington: Indiana University Press.

Petro, Jane A. and C. Andrew Salzberg. 1992. "Ethical Issues of Burn Management." *Clinics in Plastic Surgery* 19, 3 (July): 615–21.

Winslade, William. 1989. "Taken to the Limits: Pain, Identity, and Self-Transformation." In *Dax's Case: Essays in Medical Ethics and Human Meaning*, ed. Lonnie D. Kliever. Dallas: Southern Methodist University Press, 115–30.

Zawacki, Bruce E. 1989. "Tongue-Tied in the Burn Intensive Care Unit." *Critical Care Medicine* 17, 2: 198–99.

Chapter 5

The Book of the Dead. 1960. Trans. E. A. Wallis Budge. New Hyde Park, N.Y.: University Books.

Bragg, Rick. 1995. "A Cajun Christmas Tradition Won't Die Down." *New York Times,* 24 December, 10.

Brundage, Burr Cartwright. 1976. *The Phoenix of the Western World: Quetzalcoatl and the Sky Religion.* Norman: University of Oklahoma Press.

Campbell, Joseph. 1959. *The Masks of God,* Vol. 1, *Primitive Mythology.* New York: Viking.

——. 1962. *The Masks of God,* Vol. 2, *Oriental Mythology.* New York: Viking.

Cassirer, Ernst. 1946. *Language and Myth.* Trans. Suzanne Langer. New York: Harper.

Courlander, Harold and Wolf Leslain. 1995. *The Fire on the Mountain and Other Stories from Ethiopia and Eritrea.* New York: Henry Holt.

Doyle, Arthur Conan. 1894. "The Los Amigos Fiasco." In *Round the Red Lamp.* London: Methuen, 263–75.

Eliade, Mircea. 1963. *Myth and Reality.* Trans. Willard R. Trask. New York: Harper and Row.

Frazer, James George. 1922. *The Golden Bough: A Study in Religion and Magic.* Abridged ed. New York: Macmillan.

Ginzburg, Carlo. 1991. *Ecstasies: Deciphering the Witches' Sabbath.* Trans. Raymond Rosenthal. New York: Penguin.

Herodotus. 1943. The *History of Herodotus.* Trans. George Rawlinson. New York: Tudor.

Ovid. *Metamorphoses.* 1955. Trans. Rolfe Humphries. Bloomington: Indiana University Press.

Parinder, Geoffrey. 1967. *African Mythology.* London: Paul Hamlyn.

Spence, Basil. 1962. *Phoenix at Coventry.* New York: Harper and Row.

Strong, James. 1980. *The New Strong's Exhaustive Concordance of the Bible.* Nashville, Tenn.: Thomas Nelson.

Turner, Alice K. 1993. *History of Hell.* New York: Harcourt Brace.

Williams, Selma R. and Pamela Williams Adelman. 1978. *Riding the Nightmare: Women and Witchcraft from the Old World to Colonial Salem.* New York: HarperCollins.

Chapter 6

BOOKS

Abe, Kobo. 1966. *The Face of Another.* New York: Alfred A. Knopf.

Allen, W. S. 1951. "Weird Cremation." *True Detective,* December, p. 42.

Angle, Paul. 1946. *The Great Chicago Fire.* Chicago: Chicago Historical Society.

Arisman, Marshall. 1989. *Heaven Departed.* Tokyo: Tokyo Designers School.

Blizin, Jerry. 1951. "The Reeser Case." *St. Petersburg Times,* August 9.

Borst, Ronald V., Keith Burns, and Leith Adams. 1992. *Graven Images: The Best of Horror, Fantasy, and Science Fiction Film Art.* New York: Grove Press.

Clevely, Hugh. 1957. *Famous Fires.* New York: John Day Lo.

Connors, Martin and Julia Furtaw. 1995. *Video Hound's Golden Movie Retriever.* Detroit: Visible Ink Press.

Cromie, Robert. 1958. *The Great Chicago Fire.* New York: McGraw-Hill.

Dickens, Charles. 1852–53. *Bleak House.* Harmondsworth: Penguin, 1971.

Frank, Jeffrey. 1994. "What the Mutant Tomatoes Knew and When They Knew It." *Washington Post Weekly Edition,* January 17–23, p. 25.

Golding, William. 1979. *Darkness Visible.* New York: Harcourt Brace Jovanovich.

———. *Lord of the Flies.* 1962. New York: Coward, McCann, and Geoghegan.

Hardy, Phil. 1986. *The Encyclopedia of Horror Movies.* New York: Harper and Row.

Hersey, John. 1946. *Hiroshima.* New York: Knopf.

Kellerman, Jonathan. 1992. *Private Eyes.* New York: Bantam.

Krogman, Wilton M. 1953. "The Improbable Case of the Cinder Woman." *General Magazine and Historical Chronicle,* Winter, p. 61.

Lee, Gary. 1994. "Mushroom Clouds of Anger: Possible Radiation Subjects Jam the Hotline." *Washington Post Weekly Edition,* January 17–23, p. 1.

Leroux, Gaston. 1988. *The Phantom of the Opera.* New York: Harper Perennial.

Maclean, Norman. 1992. *Young Men and Fire.* Chicago: University of Chicago Press.

Nakazawa, Keiji. 1988. *Barefoot Gen: The Day After.* Philadelphia: New Society Publishers.

Nash, Jay Robert. 1976. *Darkest Hours.* Chicago: Nelson-Hall.

Nickell, Joe and John F. Fischer. 1984. "Spontaneous Human Combustion." *Fire and Arson Investigator* 34, 3: 4–11; 34, 4: 3–8.

———. 1987. "Incredible Cremations: Investigating Spontaneous Human Combustion Deaths." *Skeptical Inquirer* 11, 4: 352–57.

Perry, George. 1987. *The Complete Phantom of the Opera.* New York: Henry Holt.

Rossi, Jean-Baptiste (as Sebastien Japrisot). 1979. *Trap for Cinderella.* New York: Penguin.

Romm, Sharon. 1986. "Burns in Art." *Clinics in Plastic Surgery* 13: 3–8.

Ryder, Richard. 1983. "Portland's Fiery Fourth." *American History Illustrated* 18: 10–19.

Smith, Mary-Ann. 1994. *Masters of Illusion: A Novel of the Connecticut Circus Fire.* New York: Warner Books.

Stanford, Joseph. 1991. *Eyes of Prey.* New York: Putman.

FILMS

The Abominable Dr. Phibes. 1971. AIP, Great Britain. d. Robert Fuest, l.p. Vincent Price, Joseph Cotton, Terry-Thomas.

Amazing Colossal Man. 1957. d. Bert Gordon.

Backdraft. 1991. MCA. d. Ron Howard, p. Richard Lewis, l.p. Kurt Russell, Robert DeNiro, William Baldwin, Donald Sutherland.

Bambi. 1942. Disney. d. David Hand w. Larry Morey.

Batman. 1989. Warner Brothers. d. Tim Burton, l.p. Michael Keaton, Jack Nicholson, Kim Bassinger, Jack Palance, Billy Dee Williams.

Batman Forever. 1995. Warner Brothers. d. Tim Burton, l.p. Val Kilmer, Tommy Lee Jones, Jim Carrey.

The Bees. 1979. Warner Brothers. d. Alfredo Zacharias, l.p. John Carradine, John Saxon.

Blown Away. 1994. d. Stephen Hopkin, p. J. Watson, P. Denshaw, R. Lewis, l.p. Jeff Bridges, Tommy Lee Jones.

Carrie. 1976. United Artists. d. Brian DePalma, p. Paul Monash, l.p. Sissy Spacek, John Travolta, Piper Laurie.

The Climax. 1944. Universal. d/p George Waggner, l.p. Boris Karloff, Susanna Foster, Turhan Bey.

The Day After. 1983. Sultan Entertainment. d. Nicholas Meyer, l.p. Jason Robards, John Lithgow, Jo Beth Williams.

Darkman. 1990. MCA. d. Sam Raimi, l.p. Liam Neeson

Darkman II. 1994. MCA. d. Bradford May, l.p. Arnold Voslo, Larry Drake.

Die Hard. 1988. Twentieth Century Fox. d. John McTiernan, p. L. Gordon, J. Silver, l.p. Bruce Wills, Bonnie Bedelia.

The English Patient. 1997. Miramax. p. Saul Zaentz d/w Anthony Minghella l.p. Ralph Fiennes.

Eyes Without a Face (Les yeux sans visage). 1959. Champs Elysées-Lux, France. d. Georges Franju, p. Jules Borkon, l.p. Pierre Brasseur, Alida Valli.

The Face Behind the Mask. 1941. Columbia. d. Robert Florey, p. Wallace Mac Donald, l.p., Peter Lorre.

Face of Another. 1966. Teshigahara Prod. d. Hiroshi Teshigahara, w. Kobo Abe.

Fire Maidens of Outer Space. 1956. Saturn films, London. d. Cy Roth, l.p. Anthony Dexter, Susan Shaw, Paul Carpenter.

Firestarter. 1984. Universal. d. Mark Lester, p. Frank Capra, Jr, l.p. Drew Barrymore, David Keith, Heather Locklear, Martin Sheen, George C. Scott, Art Carney, Louise Fletcher.

Frankenstein. 1931. MCA d. James Whale, l.p. Boris Karloff.

Friday the Thirteenth. 1980. Paramount. d. Dean Cunningham.

Gone with the Wind. 1939. MGM

Halloween. 1978. Falcon Productions. d. John Carpenter, p. Debra Hall.

Halloween 5. 1990. Magnum Pictures, Inc. d. Dominique Othenia-Girard, p. Ramsey Thomas.

House of Wax. 1953. Warner Brothers. d. Andre Toth, p. Bryan Foy, l.p. Vincent Price, Charles Buchinski (Bronson).

Hunchback of Notre Dame. 1939. RKO. d. William Dieterle, l.p. Charles Laughton, Maureen O'Hara.

Jason Goes to Hell. 1993. New Line Cinema. d. Adam Marcus, p. Sean Cunningham (last in series of 9 "Jasons").

Man of a Thousand Faces. 1957. Universal. d. Joseph Pevney, l.p. James Cagney.

Map of the Human Heart. 1993. HBO. d/w Vincent Ward, l.p. Jason Scott Ward, John Crisodi, Jeanne Moreau.

Nightmare on Elm Street. 1984. New Line Cinema. d. Wes Craven, p. Robert Shaye, l.p. Robert Englund, Johnny Depp (with many sequels).

Nightmare on Elm Street 5: Dream Child. 1989. Media House Entertainment. l.p. Robert Englund.

The Phantom of Hollywood. 1974. MGM. d. Gene Levitt, l.p. Broderick Crawford, Peter Lawford, Jackie Coogan.

Phantom of the Opera. 1925. Universal Studio. d. Lloyd Bacon, p. Carl Laemmle, l.p. Lon Chaney, Mary Philbin.

——. 1943. Universal Studio. d. Arthur Lubin, p. George Waggner, l.p. Nelson Eddy, Susanna Foster, Claude Rains, Hume Cronyn.

——. 1955. Sono Film, Argentina. p. Carrerra.

——. 1960. Mexico. d. Fernando Cortes l.p. Tin-Tan

——. 1962. Hammer Productions, London. d. Terence Fisher, l.p. Herbert Lom, Heather Sears.

——. 1982. Columbia Artists. d. Robert Markowitz, l.p. Maximilian Schell, Jane Seymour, Michael York.

——. 1989. 21st Century Film Corp. d. Dwight Little, p. Harry Alan Towers, l.p. Robert Englund, Jill Schoelen.

Phantom of the Paradise. 1974. Pressman Williams. d. Brian DePalma, l.p. Paul Williams, William Finley, Jessica Harper.

The Queen of Outer Space. 1954. Allied Artists. d. Edward Bends, p. Ben Schwalb, l.p. Zsa Zsa Gabor.

Rocky Horror Picture Show. 1975. Fox. d. Jim Sharman, l.p. Tim Curry, Susan Sarandon, Barry Bostwick, Meatloaf.

Roxanne. 1987. Columbia Pictures. d. Fred Schepisi, w. Steve Martin, l.p. Steve Martin, Daryl Hannah, Shelly Duvall.

Schindler's List. 1993. MCA. d. Steven Spielberg, w. Steven Zaillian, l.p. Liam Neeson, Ben Kingsley, Ralph Fiennes.

Speed. 1994. Twentieth Century Fox d. Jan de Bout, p. Mark Gordon.

Tarantula. 1955. MCA. d. Jack Arnold, w. Robert M. Fresco, l.p. Leo Carroll, Clint Eastwood.

Texas Chainsaw Massacre. 1974. Vortex. d. Tobe Hooper.

Threads. 1985. British Television. d. Mike Jackson, l.p. Karen Meagher.
Them. 1954. Warner Bros. d. Gordon Douglas, l.p. James Whitmore, Fess Parker, James Arness.
Towering Inferno. 1974. Fox. d. John Guillermin, w. Sterling Silliphant, l.p. Steve McQueen, Paul Newman, William Holden, Faye Dunaway, Fred Astaire.
West Side Story. 1961. United Artists.
A Woman's Face. 1941. MGM. d. George Cukor, p. Victor Savile, l.p. Joan Crawford, Melvyn Douglas, Conrad Veidt.
Zabriskie Point. 1970. MGM. d/w Michelangelo Antonioni, l.p. Mark Frechette, Daria Halprin, Paul Fix, Rod Taylor, Harrison Ford.

Chapter 7

Benzaquin, Paul. 1959. *Holocaust: The Shocking Story of the Boston Cocoanut Grove Fire.* New York: Henry Holt.
Buck, Gurdon. 1872. "Case of Cicatricial Contractions After Burns Involving the Chin and Neck, Successfully Treated." *American Journal of the Medical Sciences* 125: 52–59.
Caldwell, Michael D. 1990. "Topical Wound Therapy—An Historical Perspective." *Journal of Trauma* 30: 116–22.
Cleghorn, D. 1792. *Medical Facts and Observations.* Vol. 2. London: Printed for J. Johnson.
Clowes, William A. 1637. *Profitable and Necessarie Booke of Observations for all Those Burnt with the Flame of Gunpowder.* 3rd ed. Reprint New York: Scholars' Facsimiles, 1945.
Cockshot, W. Paul. 1956. "The History of the Treatment of Burns." *Surgery, Gynecology and Obstetrics* 102: 16.
Davidson, E. C. 1925. "Tannic Acid in the Treatment of Burns." *Surgery, Gynecology, and Obstetrics* 41: 202–21.
Davis, J. S. 1914. *Plastic Surgery.* Philadelphia: P. Blakiston's Son and Co.
Dorsch, Walter, J. Scharff, T. Bayer, and H. Wagner. 1989. "Antiasthmatic Effects of Onion." *International Archives of Allergy and Applied Immunology* 88: 228–30.
Dorsch, Walter, Edward Schneider, T. Bayer, W. Breu, and H. Wagner. 1990. "Anti-inflammatory Effects of Onion." *International Archives of Allergy and Applied Immunology* 92: 39–42.
Fakhry, S. M., J. Alexander, D. Smith, A. A. Meyer, and H. D. Peterson. 1995. "Regional and Institutional Variation in Burn Care." *Journal of Burn Care and Rehabilitation* 16: 86–90.
Furnell, M. C. 1877. "Some Remarks on the Discovery of the Anesthetic Effects of Chloroform, and Its First Exhibition in England." *Lancet* 1: 934–38.
Gross, Samuel D. 1872. *System of Surgery.* 5th ed. Philadelphia: Henry C. Lea.
Haeger, Knut. 1988. *Illustrated History of Surgery.* New York: Bell.
Harkins, Henry N. 1942. *The Treatment of Burns.* Springfield, Ill.: Charles C. Thomas.
Hildanus, Fabricius. 1607. *De Combustionibus.* Basel.
Jones, John. 1775. *Plain Concise Practical Remarks on the Treatment of Wounds and Fractures.* New York: John Holt.
Kentish, E. 1797. *An Essay on Burns.* London.
Keyes, Robert. 1984. *Cocoanut Grove.* New York: Atheneum.
Majno, Guido. 1975. *The Healing Hand: Man and Wound in the Ancient World.* Cambridge, Mass.: Harvard University Press.
McCurdy, D. B., ed. 1906. *Chicago's Awful Theater Horror by the Survivors and Rescuers.* Chicago: Memorial Publishing Company.

Moncrief, J. A. 1971. "The Development of Topical Therapy." *Journal of Trauma* 11: 906.

Moyer, Carl A. 1953. "An Assessment of the Therapy of Burns." *Annals of Surgery* 137: 6–28.

Padgett, E. C. 1942. *Skin Grafting.* Springfield, Ill.: Charles C. Thomas.

Pernick, Martin S. 1988. *A Calculus of Suffering: Pain, Professionalism, and Anesthesia in Nineteenth-Century America.* New York: Columbia University Press.

Reverdin, J. L. 1872. "De la graeffe épidermique." *Archives of General Medicine* 19: 276.

Robotti, E. B. 1990. "The Treatment of Burns: An Historical Perspective with Emphasis on the Hand." *Hand Clinics* 6: 163–90.

Saffle, Jeffrey. 1993. "The 1942 Fire at Boston's Cocoanut Grove Nightclub." *American Journal of Surgery* 166: 581–91.

Shedd, D. P. 1958. "Historical Landmarks in the Treatment of Burns." *Surgery* 43: 1024–36.

Scarborough, J. 1983. "On Medications for Burns in Classical Antiquity." *Clinics in Plastic Surgery* 10: 603–10.

Sigerist, Henry. 1944. "Ambroise Paré's Onion Treatment of Burns." *Bulletin of Historical Medicine* 15: 143–49.

Sneve, H. 1905. "The Treatment of Burns and Skin Grafting." *Journal of the American Medical Association* 45: 1.

Stark, R. B. 1975. "The History of Plastic Surgery in Wartime." *Clinics in Plastic Surgery* 2: 509–16.

Tagliacozzi, Gaspare. 1597. *De curatorum chirurgia.* Venice: Robertus Meiettus.

Underhill, Frank P. 1930. "The Significance of Anhydremia in Extensive Surface Burn." *Journal of the American Medical Association* 95: 852.

Wallace, A. F. 1987. "Recent Advances in the Treatment of Burns — 1843–1858." *British Journal of Plastic Surgery* 40: 193–200.

Wiseman, Richard. 1676. *Severrall Chirurgical Treatises.* London.

Chapter 8

Allen, H. S. and S. L. Koch. 1942. "The Treatment of Patients with Severe Burns." *Surgery, Gynecology, Obstetrics* 79: 914.

Artz, Curtis Price. 1969. "Burns in My Lifetime." *Journal of Trauma* 9: 827–33.

Beard, Jonathan. 1994. "Fresh Approach to a Familiar Problem: Skin Replacement." *New York Times,* 30 January.

Benmeir, P., A. Sagi, B. Greber, et al. 1991. "An Analysis of Mortality in Patients with Burns Covering 40% BSA or More: A Retrospective Review Covering 24 Years (1964–88)." *Burns* 17: 402ff..

Bernstein, Norman. 1976. *Emotional Problems of the Facially Burned and Disfigured.* Boston: Little, Brown.

Blakeney, P., D. Herndon and M. Desar. 1988. "Long-Term Psychosocial Adjustment Following Burn Injuries." *Journal of Burn Care and Rehabilitation* 9: 661–65.

Bowder, M. L. and I. Feller. 1985. "Disfigurement and Body Images as Variables in Adaption of the Burn Injury." *Bulletin and Clinical Review of Burn Injuries* 7: 36.

Brown, J. B. and McDowell, F. 1942. "Massive Repairs of Burns with Thick Split-Skin Grafts." *Annals of Surgery* 115: 658.

Brown, J. B., M. P. Fryer, P. Randall, and M. Lu. 1953. "Post-Mortem Homografts as Biological Dressings for Extensive Burns and Denuded Areas." *Annals of Surgery* 138: 618.

Burke, J. F., C. C. Bondoc, and W. C. Quinby. 1976. "Primary Burn Excision and Immediate Grafting: A Method of Shortening Illness. *Journal of Trauma* 14: 389.

Cairns, B. A., S. deSerres, H. D. Peterson, and A. A. Meyer. 1993. "Skin Replacements: The Biotechnological Quest for Optimal Wound Closure." *Archives of Surgery* 128: 1249.

Cianci, P. and R. Sato. 1994. "Adjuvant Hyperbaric Oxygen Therapy in the Treatment of Thermal Burns: A Review." *Burns* 20: 5–14.

Cobb, M., G. Maxwell, and P. Silvestri. 1990. "Patient Perception of Quality of Life After Burn Injury: Results of an 11-Year Survey." *Journal of Burn Care and Rehabilitation* 11: 330–33.

Colebrook, L., T. Gibson, and J. P. Todd. 1945. *Studies of Burns and Scalds.* Medical Research Council Special Report Series 249. London: HMSO.

Dimick, A. R., P. A. Brigham, and E. M. Sheehy. 1993. "The Development of Burn Centers in North America." *Journal of Burn Care and Rehabilitation* 14: 284–99.

Davidson, E. C. 1926. "The Prevention of Toxemia of Burns: Treatment by Tannic Acid Solution." *American Journal of Surgery* 40: 114.

Doctor, Marion E. 1992. "Burn Camps and Community Aspects of Burn Care." *Journal of Burn Care and Rehabilitation* 13, 1: 68–76.

Dunbar, J. 1934. "Review of Burn Cases treated in the Glasgow Royal Infirmary During the Past Hundred Years (1833–1933), with some Observations on the Present-Day Treatment." *Glasgow Medical Journal* 122: 239–55.

Dziewulski, P. 1991. "Burn Wound Healing: James Ellsworth Laing Memorial Essay for 1991." *Burns* 18:466.

Eisenberg, Mark. 1987. "Successful Engraftment of Cultured Human Epidermal Autograft." *Medical Journal of Australia* 147: 520–21.

Eyles, P., G. Browne and C. Byrne. 1984. "Methodological Problems in Studies of Burn Survivors and Their Psychosocial Prognosis." *Burns* 10: 427–33.

Feller, I., D. Tholen, and R. G. Cornell. 1980. "Improvements in Burn Care, 1965–1979." *Journal of the American Medical Association* 244: 2074–78.

Feller, I. and C. A. Jones. 1987. "The National Burn Information Exchange: The Use of a National Burn Registry to Evaluate and Address the Burn Problem." *Surgical Clinics of North America* 67: 167–89.

Fox, C. L. 1968. "Silver Sulfadiazine — A New Topical Therapy for Pseudomonas in Burns." *Archives of Surgery* 96: 184.

Gallico, G. G., N. E. O'Connor, C. C. Compton, O. Kehinde, and H. Green. 1984. "Permanent Coverage of Large Burn Wounds with Autologous Cultured Human Epithelium." *New England Journal of Medicine* 311: 448.

Gibson, T. 1955. "Zoografting — A Curious Chapter in the History of Plastic Surgery." *British Journal of Plastic Surgery* 8: 234.

Green, H., O. Kehinde, and J. Thomas. 1979. "Growth of Cultured Human Epidermal Cells into Multiple Epithelia Suitable for Grafting." *Proceedings of the National Academy of Science in the U.S.A.* 76: 5665.

Harkins, Henry N. 1942. "The Treatment of Burns in Wartime." *Journal of the American Medical Association* 119: 385.

Heimbach, D. M. 1987. "Early Burn Excision and Grafting." *Surgical Clinics of North America* 67: 93–107.

Helm, Phala A. 1992. "Burn Rehabilitation: Dimensions of the Problem." *Clinics in Plastic Surgery* 19: 551–59.

Jackson, D. M. 1991. "The Evolution of Burn Treatment in the Last 50 Years." *Burns* 17: 329.

Janzekovic, A. Z. 1970. "A New Concept in the Early Excision and Immediate Grafting of Burns." *Journal of Trauma* 10: 1103.

Jie, X. and C. B. Ren. 1992. "Burn Injuries in the Dong Bei Area of China: A Study of 12,606 Cases." *Burns* 18.

Knighton, D. R., B. Halliday and T. K. Hunt. 1984. "Oxygen as an Antibiotic: The Effect of Inspired Oxygen on Infection. *Archives of Surgery* 119: 199.

MacGregor, F. C. 1953. *Facial Deformities and Plastic Surgery: A Psychosocial Study.* Springfield, Ill.: Charles C. Thomas.

MacIndoe, A. H. 1940. "The Functional Aspect of Burn Therapy." *Proceedings of the Royal Society of Medicine* 34: 56.

MacMillan, Bruce G. 1974. "No Man Ever Stands so Tall . . . ." *Journal of Trauma* 14: 731–42.

Moncrief, J. A. and J. A. Rivera. 1958. "The Problem of Infection in Burns by Resistant Micro-Organisms with a Note on the Use of Bacitracin. *"Annals of Surgery* 147: 295.

Moyer, C. A., L. Brentano, D. Gravens, et al. 1965. "Treatment of Large Burns with 0.5% Silver Nitrate Solution." *Archives of Surgery* 90: 812.

Niu, A. K. C., C. Yang, and H. C. Lee. 1987. "Burns Treated with Adjunctive Hyperbaric Oxygen Therapy: A Comparative Study in Humans." *Journal of Hyperbaric Medicine* 2: 75.

O'Connor, N. E, J. B. Milliken, S. Banks-Schlegel, O. Kehinde, and H. Green. 1981. "Grafting of Burns with Cultured Epithelium Prepared from Autologous Epidermal Cells." *Lancet:* 75.

Pack, G. T. and A.H. Davis. 1930. *Burns.* Philadelphia: Lippincott.

Peters, W. J. 1980. "Biological Dressing in Burns — A Review." *Annals of Plastic Surgery* 4: 133–37.

Petro, J. A. and C.A. Salzburg. 1992. "Ethical Issues of Burn Management." *Clinics in Plastic Surgery* 19: 615–21.

Prasad, J. K., M. L. Bowder, and P. H. Thomson. 1991. "A Review of the Reconstructive Surgery Needs of 3,126 Survivors of Burn Injury." *Burns* 17: 302–5.

Pruzinsky, T., L. D. Rice, H. N. Himel, R. F. Morgan, and R. F. Edlich. 1992. "Psychometric Assessment of Psychologic Factors Influencing Adult Burn Rehabilitation." *Journal of Burn Care and Rehabilitation* 13: 79–88.

Pollock, G. D. 1871. "Cases of Skin Grafting and Transplantation." *Transactions of the Clinical Society of London* 4: 375.

Reig, A., C. Tejerina, P. Baena, and V. Mirabet. 1994. "Massive Burns: a Study of Epidemiology and Mortality." *Burns* 20: 51.

Rheinwald, J. G. and H. Green. 1975. "Serial Cultivation of Strains of Human Epidermal Keratinocytes: The Formation of Keratinizing Colonies from Single Cells. *Cell* 6: 331.

Robson, M. C., T.J. Krizek, N. Koss, et al. 1973. "Amniotic Membrane as a Temporary Wound Dressing." *Surgery, Gynecology, Obstetrics* 136: 787.

Salisbury, R. 1992. "Burn Rehabilitation: Our Unanswered Challenge. *"Journal of Burn Care and Rehabilitation* 13: 495–505.

Sheffield, C. G., G. B. Irons, P. Mucha, et al. 1988. "Physical and Psychological Outcomes After Burns." *Journal of Burn Care and Rehabilitation* 9: 172–77.

Silvetti, A. N., C. Cotlon, and R. J. Byrne. 1957. "Preliminary Experimental Studies of Bovine Embryo Skin Grafts." *Transplantation Bulletin* 4: 25.

Stark, Richard B. 1975. "The History of Plastic Surgery in Wartime." *Clinics in Plastic Surgery* 2: 509–16.

Subrahmanyam, M. 1994. "Honey-Impregnated Gauze Versus Amniotic Membrane in the Treatment of Burns." *Burns* 20: 331–33.

Sutton, G. 1993. "Entry to the Burn Team: Stressors, Supports, and Coping Strategies." *Burns* 19, 4: 349–51.

Tanner, J. C., J. Vandeput and J. F. Olley. 1964. "The Mesh Graft." *Plastic and Reconstructive Surgery* 34: 287.

Topley, E. 1961. "The Usefulness of Counting 'Heat-Affected' Red Cells as a Guide to the Risk of Late Disappearance of Red Cells After Burns." *Journal of Clinical Pathology* 10: 1.

Underhill, Frank P. 1930. "The Significance of Anhydrosis in Extensive Superficial Burns." *Journal of the American Medical Association* 96: 833.

Venable, A. 1914. "The Use of Pig Skin in Extensive Grafts." *Southwestern Journal of Medicine and Surgery* 22: 341–45.

Chapter 9

Doctor, Marion E. 1992. "Burn Camps and Community Aspects of Burn Care." *Journal of Burn Care and Rehabilitation* 13, 1: 68–76.

The Guinea Pig Club. 1991. (film). Aviation Classics Limited.

Korte, Melinda A., Stephanie Daniels, and C. Wayne Cruse. 1990. "A Description of Recreation Therapy Services in the Burn Unit. Abstract. *Proceedings of the American Burn Association* 142.

Mahaney, Nancy Bell. 1990. "Restoration of Play in a Severely Burned Three-Year-Old Child." *Journal of Burn Care and Rehabilitation* 11, 1: 57–63.

Pruzinsky, Thomas, Linda Rice, Harvey N. Himel, Raymond F. Morgan, and Richard F. Edlich. 1992. "Psychometric Assessment of Psychologic Factors Influencing Adult Burn Rehabilitation." *Journal of Burn Care and Rehabilitation* 13: 79–88.

Sheffield, Charles G., George B. Irons, Peter Mucha Jr., et al. 1988. "Physical and Psychological Outcomes After Burns." *Journal of Burn Care and Rehabilitation* 9: 171–77.

Chapter 10

America Burning: Report of the National Commission of Fire Prevention and Control. 1973. Washington, D.C.: U.S. Government Printing Office.

America Burning: Revisited. 1988. U.S. Fire Administration, Federal Emergency Management Agency. Washington, D.C.: U.S. Government Printing Office.

Botkin, J. R. 1988. "The Fire-Safe Cigarette." *Journal of the American Medical Association* 260: 226–29.

Byrd, Lee Merrill. "Major Six Pockets." In *My Sister Disappears: Stories and a Novella.* Dallas: Southern Methodist University Press, 15–39.

Carter, Albert Howard, III. 1995. "Self-Help." *Encyclopedia of Bioethics*, rev. ed., ed. Warren T. Reich. New York: Macmillan.

Feller, I. and C. A. Jones. 1987. "The National Burn Information Exchange: The Use of a National Burn Registry to Evaluate and Address the Burn Problem." *Surgical Clinics of North America* 67: 167–89.

Mapp, Louise, David G. Greenhalgh, J. Richard Kagan, and Glenn D. Warden. 1993. "A Nationwide Survey of Burn Recovery and Support Groups." Abstract. *Proceedings of the American Burn Association* 25: 181.

Munster, A. M., M. Smith-Meek, and P. Sharkey. 1994. "The Effect of Early Surgical Intervention on Mortality and Cost-Effectiveness in Burn Care." *Burn* 20, 1: 515–20.

Peet, Walter J., Cindy K. Leenknecht, Vera Reineking, and Barbara Sherman. 1993. "The Development and Support of a Regional Burn Team." Abstract. *Proceedings of the American Burn Association* 25: 183.

Sacks, J. J. and D. E. Nelson. 1994. "Smoking and Injuries: An Overview." *Preventive Medicine* 23, 4: 515–20.

Silverstein, P. and B. Lack. 1987. "Fire Prevention in the United States: Are the Home Fires Still Burning?" *Surgical Clinics of North America* 67: 1.

Sutton, G. 1993. "Entry to the Burn Team: Stressors, Supports, and Coping Strategies." *Burns* 19, 4: 349–51.

Turner, Dale G. and Cheryl J. Leman. 1989. "Cooking-Related Burn Injuries in the Elderly: Preventing the 'Granny Gown' Burn." Abstract. *Proceedings of the American Burn Association* 21: 152.

White, Barbara J. and Edward Madara. 1995. *The Self-Help Source Book.* 5th ed. Denville, N.J.: Northwest Covenant Medical Center.

White, W. V. 1971. "Flammable Fabrics and the Burn Problem: A Status Report." *American Journal of Public Health* 61: 20–57.

Wiley, Robert G. 1993. "Trauma/Burn Seminars for Clergy: An Approach to Healing and Restoration for Burn Patients and Their Families." Abstract. *Proceedings of the American Burn Association* 25: 186.

Epilogue

Camus, Albert. 1946. *The Plague.* Trans. Stuart Gilbert. New York: Random House, 1972.

Schanke, Robert A. 1992. *Shattered Applause: The Lives of Eva Le Gallienne.* Carbondale and Edwardsville: Southern Illinois University Press.

"Spotlight on Our Members." 1966. *Icarus File* 11, 2 (Winter-Spring): 18–19.

Appendix 2

Bare, William K. 1977. *Fundamentals of Fire Prevention.* New York: John Wiley and Sons.

——. 1978. *Introduction to Fire Science and Fire Protection.* New York: John Wiley and Sons.

Roblee, Charles L., Allen J. McKechnie, and William Lundy. 1981. *The Investigation of Fires.* Englewood Cliffs, N.J.: Prentice-Hall.

Index

Note: Page numbers in italics refer to figures. The term "passim" indicates that relevant information is found throughout a chapter.

Abe, Kobo, 123
Abominable Dr. Phibes, The (film), 203
absolute zero, 41
absurdity, 48
accidental burns, 25, 37–38, 56–58
acid burns, 59, 60, 122, 123
acids. *See* battery acid; picric acid; tannic acid
"acting out," burns as, 26–27
Adamanese mythology, 94
adenosine triphosphate (ATP), 40
adrenaline, 14
age, and survivorship, 178
Agni, 92–93, 100
AIDS, 55
Ainu mythology, 96
air-flotation beds, 73
alcohol, as burn treatment, 138
alcohol fuel, burns from, 59, 82
alcoholism, 55
Allen, H. S., 165
allopathic medicine, 141, 142
Amazing Colossal Man (film), 119
America Burning, 188, 189
America Burning Revisited, 188
American Burn Association, 29, 171, 173, 176, 194
American Indians. *See* Native Americans
amniotic membranes, as biological dressings, 159
amputation, 50, 53
anesthesia, 140–41
Ansari, Saeed A., 44
antibiotics, 167
antisepsis, 140, 141, 164
apocalyptic imagery, 63, 104

Arabic gum, 133
arborescent erythema, 24
Arisman, Marshall, 128, *129*
Aristotle, 133
Armageddon, fear of, 33
arson: detection of, 187; potential for burns from, 60, 63
art, fire and burn imagery in, 128–30
artificial skin, 155, 158–59
Arturson, C., 2
Artz, Curtis, 189
Assyrian mythology, 91
asymmetrical relationships, 29
attacks, burns in, 60
Auden, W. H., 101
autografts, 155, 160, 161
autologous blood, 162–63
auto mechanics, risk of burns for, 45
autopsies, 178
Aztec mythology, 92

Backdraft (film), 39, 89, 119, 120
Ballingall, Sir George, 139
Baltimore, fire in, 125
Bambi (film), 119, 120
barbecue coals, burns from, 36, 42, 44, 58, 82
Barefoot Gen: The Day After (Nakazawa), 124
Batman, imagery of, 109, 113, 118. *See also* Joker
battery acid, burns from, 59
Baxter, Charles, 154
Bees, The (film), 120
beeswax, 157. *See also* honeycomb
Beffa, Harvey, 189
Beltane fires, 100

Benin mythology, 92
Bently, J. Irving, 121
benu bird, *103*
Bernstein, Norman, 174
betrayal: fear of, 32; following burn incident, 46–49, 55
Bible (New Testament): eschatological passages in, 39; fire of Holy Spirit in, 96, 99; references to fires and burning in, 96–97
Biliku, 94
bioethics, 75, 80
biological dressings, 156–59
Blair, Vilray, 143
Blakeney, P., 174
Bleak House (Dickens), 120–21
Blocker, Truman, 165
blood replacement (transfusions), 154, 162–64
Blown Away (film), 110, 120
blue-collar workers, risk of burns for, 45
Blumenfield, Michael, 14, 54, 55, 82
body: fear of damage to, 32; loss of parts of, 50, 53. *See also* amputation; disfigurement
body temperature, regulation of, 40–41, 51
boiling water, burns from, 42, 59. *See also* hot water; scald burns
bones: damage to, 18, 53–54, 73; loss of density, 54
bonfires, 100–101, 104
Boston City Hospital, 146, 147
Botkin, J. R., 189
Bowder, M. L., 174
bra burning, 100
Branch Davidians, 63
Brazil: burns in, 44, 151; burn treatment in, 159
Breslau, Alan Jeffry, 7, 22, 27, 103, 184
Bringgold, Diane, 22
Brooke Army Hospital (San Antonio, Tex.), 39, 152, 175, 189
Browder, Newton, 147
Brown, James Barrett, 143, 157
Brown, Larry, 13–14, 29
Brueghel, Pieter (the Elder), 101, 102
Brundage, Burr Cartwright, 103
Buck, Gurdon, 131
Buddha, 93–94
Buddhist monks, self-immolation of, 62, 63, *107*, 107–8
building codes, 188
Burke, J. F., 155

burn beds: definition of, 151; numbers of, 176
burn camps, 175, 184, 196
burn care. *See* burn treatments
burn-care personnel. *See* caregivers
burn centers: definition of, 151; funding of, 176, 189; location of, 171, 180; treatment in, 152–54. *See also* burn units
burn delirium, 55, 170
burn illness, natural history of, 138
burn infection. *See* infections
burn patients: blaming, 6; burns defined by, 22–27; helplessness of, 33, 67, 81; limitations imposed on, 65–85 passim; metabolic status of, 17; motivation of, 24, 182, 184; as prisoners, 29, 66–85; psychological status of, 54–56, 81–84, 173–74, 182–85; rebelliousness of, 25, 67, 73; responses to extremity, 15; rituals of, 25–26; self-images of, 25; visiting of, 77, 78–79
burn rounds, participants in, 28, 79, 194–95
burns: ascribed (symbolic) meaning of, 6, 50; caregivers' definition of, 28–30; causes (agents) of, 16, 17–18, 36–49 passim, 64; contemporary imagery of, 105–30 passim; as defined by fears, 31–34; definition of, 11–35 passim, 50; degrees (levels) of, 16, 18–19, 136, 138, 139; duration of, 25; extent (area and depth) of, 18–19; family and friends' definition of, 27–28; incidence of, 190; medical consequences ("sequelae") of, 50–56; medical definition of, 16–21; metaphoric meanings of, 30–31; myths about, 89–104 passim; pain associated with, 17, 22; patients' definition of, 22–27; physicality of, 11; prevention of, 152, 186–89, 192; surgical treatment of, 142–43; treatment of wounds by, 134–35; visibility of, 18
burn salves, 165–67
burn shock, 17, 50, 52, 142, 145, 146
Burns United Support Group, 196
burn survivors: focus on causes of their burns, 58; imagery of, 6–7; impairment of, 173; long–term experiences of, 4, 177, 179–85; memoirs of, 124–27; psychological status of, 182–85; re-entry into public world by, 25, 77–78; rehabilitation of, 151, 152, 169–75; support groups for, 195; transformation of, 26, 58, 184
burn treatments: costs of, 173, 174–75, 180, 192; history of, 131–47 passim; maggot

therapy, 161–62; modern, 151–76 passim, 189–90; participants in, 168–69, 193–95; pressure therapy, 69–73, *72*, 137, 172; problems in, 191–93; purpose of, 151–52; recommendations for, 197–98; strengths of, 193–96; whole-person approach, 193. *See also* debridement; infections; skin grafts

burn units: declining number of, 176; definition of, 151; "imprisonment" in, 66–85; isolation of, 14, 77; mirrors in, 24; as "nursery", 67, 81; temperature of, 13, 51; transfer to, 74–75. *See also* burn centers

cadavers, skin grafts from, 159, 161
Cagney, James, 202
Cain, imagery of, 13, 31, 38
Cajun traditions, 100–101
Campbell, Joseph, 91, 92, 93, 94
campfires, 104
Camus, Albert, 199
Canaday, 156
candles, symbolism associated with, 104
capital punishment, 98
Captain Ahab, imagery of, 31, 43
carbon monoxide, 189
carburetor burns, 45
caregivers: burns defined by, 28–30; motivation of, 14, 28–29; responses to extremity, 13–15. *See also* medical profession
Carrie (film), 119, 120, 121
carron oil, as burn treatment, 139, 143
castor oil, as burn treatment, 157
cells, levels of damage to, 19
Celsus, 133, 134.138
Challenger explosion, 33
Chaney, Lon, 111, *112*, 202–3
chaplains, as caregivers, 28, 84
charcoal fires. *See* barbecue coals
chemical burns, 17
chemical restraints (medications), 73, 79–80
Chernobyl disaster, 152
Chicago, Great Fire of, 124, 125–27
child abuse, burns as, 59–60
children: burning of, 59–60; recovery of, 184; treatment of, 76–77, *77*
China: burn mortality rates in, 151; fire mythology of, 92; prehistoric fires in, 90
chloroform anesthesia, 140
Choukoutien Cave, 90
Christian Science, 142
Christian symbolism, 99–101. *See also* Bible (New Testament)

cicatrization, 139
cigarette (and cigar) burns, 59, 60, 188–89
Cigarette Safety Act of 1984, 189
Clark, Brian C., 73
Cleghorn, David, 137, 138, 139
Climax, The (film), 202
clothes irons, burns from, 36
clothing, flammability standards for, 189
Clowes, William, 136
coals, barbecue. *See* barbecue coals
Cobb, M., 174
Cocoanut Grove fire (Boston), 146, 147, 152
Cold War, fear of nuclear confrontation during, 39
Colebrook, Leonard, 165
Commission on Fire Prevention and Control, 188
compression garments, *72*, 172
conduction, 205
contact burns, 1
contractures, *70–71*, 111, 113, 136–37, 139, 140, *141*, 142, 171, 181. *See also* scar tissue
control, fear of loss of, 33
convection, 205
cooking, accidents during, 57, 82, 186
cooking fires. *See* open fires
cooking oil, burns from, 42
cooking pots, proper placement of handles of, 46
Coover, Robert, 33
Cope, Oliver, 147, 154
copper sulfate, as burn treatment, 133, 134, 165
cosmetic surgery, 175, 180
Cowart, Dax, 29, 69, 80, 83, 198
Crane, Stephen, 12–13, 23, 34, 43, 105
Crawford, Joan, 201
cremation, 40, 53, 61
cultured skin, 155, 160–61
Cyrano de Bergerac, 108

Daedalus, imagery of, 38, 101–2
Dante Alighieri, 43, 98
Darkman (film), imagery of, 12, 34, 73, 105, 108, 109, 114–15, *116*, *117*, 117–18, 204
Darkness Visible (Golding), 122–23
Davidson, Edward, 143–44, 165
Davis, John Staige, 143
Day After, The (film), 39
Day of Wrath ("Dies Irae"), 33
death: desire for, 82; fear of, 32, 79, 82–83. *See also* mortality rate

debridement, 29, 68–69, 75, 155
deep partial thickness burns, definition of, 19
deformities, imagery of, 108–9
DeKetham, Johannes, 133
denaturing, of skin cells, 19
DeNiro, Robert, 120
dermatome, 143, *144*, 155, 159
dermis: damage to, 18; preservation of, 156
de Vigo, Giovanni, 134, 135
devil, imagery of, 12
diabetes, 55
Dickens, Charles, 120–21
Die Hard (film), 110, 120
disability, versus impairment, 173
disability benefits, 26, 169, 173
disasters, problems handling, 191
disfigurement: fear of, 31; patients' reactions to, 22, 23, 173–74
Doctor, Marion, 184
Dr. Doom, 108
Dogon mythology, 92
Dorsch, Walter, 136
Doyle, Arthur Conan, 98
Dresden, destruction of, 39, 61, 124
Dunbar, J., 164
Dupont Plaza Hotel fire (Puerto Rico), 188
Duppa, Darell, 103
Dupuytren, Guillaume, 18, 138, 139

early excision, 156
Ebers Papyrus, 132, 156
Edwards, Jonathan, 98
effigies, burning of, 100
Egyptian burn treatments, 132–33, 156
Ehrlich, Gretel, 24
Eisenberg, Mark, 160
elastic garments, 69–73, *72*
elder-oil, as burn treatment, 135
electrical energy: potential for burns from, 18, 36, 37; severity of injury from, 53, 54, 179
electric chair, 98
electrocution, 97–98
emergency medical system, 74, 191
emergency rooms, 74
emergency workers, responses to extremity, 13–14
enemas, 137
English Patient, The (Ondaatje), 34
Englund, Robert, *114*, 204
epidermis, damage to, 18

epidermolysis bullosa congenita (EBC), 18, 160
epilepsy, 82
epithelialization, 139
EPO-erythropoeitin (Epogen (R)), 155
eroticism, and burning metaphors, 30–31
eschar, 19, 67, 143
escharotomy, 67, *68*
eschaton, 33, 39
Esslin, Martin, 48
ether anesthesia, 140
Ethiopia: fire mythology of, 95; prehistoric fires in, 90
euthanasia, 80
exchange transfusions, 154
extremity: as context for burns, 11; examination of, 5–7; medical responses to, 13–15; traditional cultural interpretations of, 12–13
Eyes of Prey (Stanford), 122
Eyes Without a Face (film), 203
Eyles, P., 172

fabrics, flammability standards for, 189
Face Behind the Mask, The (film), 201
Face of Another, The (Abe), 123
Fakhry, S. M., 132
fall, myths of, 94, 101–2
family: burns defined by, 27–28; as caregivers, 195; difficulty in recognizing burn patients, 75; visits by, 77, 78–79
Fantasma de la Operta, El (film), 202
Fantastic Four super heroes, 118
fears, burn patients defined by, 31–34
Federal Emergency Management Agency, 189
Feller, Irving, 174, 190
fertility rites, fire associated with, 99–100
fiery furnace, imagery of, 96–97, 113
fiery serpents, imagery of, 97
films, burn imagery in, 110–20, 121, 201–4
fire: behavior of, 119–20, 205–6; modern symbolic rituals of, 99–101; myths about, 89–104 passim; prehistoric uses of, 90–91; used as military weapon, 60, 61
fire detectors, 187
firefighters, support for burn centers from, 190, 198
firefighting equipment, 125
fire-giving myths, 91–95
Fire Maidens of Outer Space (film), 202
firemaking tools, prehistoric, 90

fireplaces, value of, 104
Fire Prevention Week, 187
fires. *See* arson; bonfires; campfires; fire;
   open fires
Fire Sermon, 93–94
Firestarter (film), 121
fire-taking myths, 91–95
fireworks, burns from, 43, 44
first-degree burns, 16, 18, 139
flag burning, 100
flame burns, 1, 44
flaming, 205, 206
flash burns, 1
flash-overs, 205, 206
fluid replacement, 145, 147, 154–55
Fluosol, 163–64
food: burn patients' need for, 53, 167–68;
   burns from, 58–59, 82. *See also* cooking,
   accidents during
foot contracture, *70–71*
forest fires, burns from, 36, 43
four elements, 90
fourth-degree burns, 18
Fox, Charles L., 166
Franju, Georges, 203
Frankenstein (film), 120
Frankenstein (Shelley), 12–13
Frankenstein's monster, imagery of, 12, 102,
   105, 109, 117
fraternities, burns as initiation rites in, 63
Frazer, James George, 91, 94, 99, 100
Freddy Krueger, imagery of, 12, 89, 108, 109,
   113, *114*
friction burns, 17
Friday the Thirteenth (film), 113
friends: burns defined by, 27–28; as caregivers, 195–96; difficulty in recognizing
   burn patients, 75; visits by, 77, 78–79
frog skin, 159
frostbite, burns from, 17, 41
Fuji (fire goddess), 92, 96
Fuji, Mount, 96
full thickness burns: definition of, 19; pain
   associated with, 31
functionality, fear of loss of, 31–32
Furnell, M. C., 140
furniture fires, 188, 189

Gabor, Zsa Zsa, 202
Galen, 90, 133, 134, 138
Gallico, G. G., 160
gasoline, burns from, 45, 56–57, 153

geothermal energy, burns from, 40
geysers, burns from, 36, 40
Gibil, 91
Gilles, H. D., 131, 175
"glove" burns, 60
glowing, 205
Goffman, Erving, 33
Golding, William, 122–23
Gone with the Wind (film), 39
Götterdämmerung, 33, 39, 99
"granny gown burns," 186
granulation, 142
Grealy, Lucy, 22, 23
grease: burns from, 42, 47; as burn treat-
   ment, 134
Greek mythology, 91–92, 96, 101–2
Green, H., 160
Gross, Samuel, 131
guilt, fear of, 32–33
Guinea Pig Club, 185
gunpowder, burns from, 58, 131, 134, 136
Guyon, Félix Jacques, 142

Hades, 98
hair removal wax, burns from, 43
Halloween, 100
Halloween (film), 113
Hamlet (N.C.) chicken processing plant fire,
   188
Happyland Social Club fire (Bronx), 188
Harkins, Henry N., 154
Harry "Two-Faced" Dent, 118
Hartford Circus disaster, 122
Harvard Medical School, 160
healing. *See* burn patients; burn survivors;
   burn treatments
health-care surrogacy, 179
hearths: gods of, 91–92; prehistoric, 90; symbolism of, 96
heat: cultural meanings of, 43–45; definition
   of, 40–42; in fires, 206
heat exhaustion, 41
heating pads, burns from, 43
heat sources: burns from, 11, 17, 36–37, 38–
   43; description of, 38–40, 42–43
heat stroke, 41, 51
Heaven Departed (Arisman), 128
Hell: fear of, 33; imagery of, 43, 98–99
helplessness, fear of, 33
Hephaestus, 91, 92
heretics, burning of, 97
Herodotus, 102–3, 133

Hersey, John, 124
Hestia, 91–92, 96
heterografts (xenografts), 155, 156, 158
heterotrophic bone formation, 180
Heyfelder, Oskar, 140
high-rise buildings, fires in, 49
high-risk behaviors, burns from, 58
high-voltage electricity. *See* electrical energy
Hildanus, Fabricius, 135, 136
Hill, Ken, 115
Hindu skin grafting, 142
Hippocrates, 134
Hiroshima (Hersey), 124
Hiroshima, destruction of, 39, 104, 124
Holocaust: fires associated with, 61, 104;
    theological questions about, 55
homeless people, survival rate of, 26
homeostasis, 51
homografts, 155, 156–58
honey, as burn treatment, 133, 134, 159,
    165
honeycomb, 133, 134. *See also* beeswax
Hornby, 137
hot springs, burns from, 40
hot water, burns from, 59, 60, 186–87. *See also*
    boiling water; hot springs; scald burns
House of Wax (film), 120, 202
Howland, George, 126–27
Hubbard tanks, 29, 69, 83, 155
Human Torch, 118
Hutchinson, Jonas, 126
hyperbaric oxygen, 163
hypermetabolism, 53, 138
hypertrophic scars, 31, 69, *70–71*, 181
Hypocrites, 134
hypothermia, 41, 51

Icarus, imagery of, 6, 38, 101–2, 102, 177
Icarus File, The (newsletter), 195
"ICU psychosis," 55
Ila mythology, 92
image, definition of, 23–24
imagination, influence on healing, 24
Imbus, Sharon, 80
immune system, response to burn, 52–53
Impact (Arisman), 128, *129*
impairment, versus disability, 173
Incan mythology, 92
incendiary bombs, burns from, 42
incense: burns from, 63; as burn treatment,
    133
India: burning of women in, 60, 61–62; burn

treatment in, 44, 159; Vedic mythology of,
    92–93, 100
infections, 17, 50, 52–53, 77, 134, 138, 146,
    159, 164–67
Inferno (Dante), 43, 98
inhalation injuries, 42, 54, 147, 170, 178
injury: definition of, 17; psychological, 46–
    49, 54–56, 81–84, 173–74, 182–85
insult, definition of, 24
intentional burns, 25, 58–63. *See also* suicide
    attempts, failed
Iroquois Theater fire (Chicago), 146

Jackson, D. M., 164
Janzekovic, A. Zora, 155–56
Japanese mythology, 92
Jason, imagery of, 113
J.B. (MacLeish), 55
Jehovah's Witnesses, 153, 162
Jesus of Nazareth, 102
jet fuel, burns from, 36
Jewish mythology, 93
Joan of Arc, 97
Job, story of, 55
Jobst, Inc., 72
Jobst garments, 72, 172, 174–75
Johnny Tremain, 31
joints, scar tissue over, 54. *See also* contracture
Joker, 105, 108, 113
Jones, John, 138–39
Joyce, James, 98

Karloff, Boris, 202
Kashmir, burns in, 44
Kaska mythology, 94
Kehinde, O., 160
Kellerman, Jonathan, 122
Keneally, Thomas, 61
Kentish, Edward, 137, 138, 139
Kenya, prehistoric fires in, 90
Kevorkian, Jack, 80
Kids on the Block program, 184
kinetic molecular theory, 40
King, Aurelia, 127
Koch, S. L., 165
Koresh, David, 63
Krause, Charles J., 143
Kushner, Harold S., 55

Lactanius, 102
lactated Ringer's solution, 153, 154
Laemmle, Carl, 111

lanolin, as burn treatment, 157
Lawrence (saint), 97, 108
Lawrence, D. H., 103
Le Gallienne, Eva, 198
Leroux, Gaston, 110, 111, 115
lesion, definition, 17
Levinson, Stanley M., 147
Lifton, Robert J., 61
lighter fluid, burns from, 42, 57
lightning, burns from, 24, 36, 40, 43
Lightning Strike and Electric Shock Victims
    International Group, 196
lime water, as burn treatment, 139
Lindberg, Robert, 166
Lindsay, 166
linseed oil, as burn treatment, 139, 143
liquified petroleum gas explosions, 2
Lister, Joseph, 141, 164
Liston, Robert, 140
living wills, 75, 179
Loki, 92
Lom, Herbert, 203
London, Great Fire of, 124
Lord of the Flies (Golding), 122
Lorre, Peter, 201
Lund, Charles
Lund-Browder chart, 18, *20*, 147
lung failure, 54
lye, burns from, 59

MacGregor, Frances, 173
MacIndoe, Archibald, 131, 143, 165, 185
Maclean, Norman, 40, 124
MacLeish, Archibald, 55
maggot therapy, 161–62
Mahayana tradition (Japanese Buddhism),
    63
Maher, Ellen L., 31
Majno, Guido, 133
Man of a Thousand Faces (film), 202–3
Map of the Human Heart (film), 61
Martin, Steve, 98, 108
Mason, Warren, 142
Massachusetts General Hospital, 146, 147
Masters of Illusion (Smith), 122
Maugham, Somerset, 108
May, William F., 25, 81
Mayo Clinic, 174
McAuliffe, Christy, 33
McDonald, Edward D., 103
McDowell, F., 157
meaning, types of, 15–16

Medical College of Virginia, 175
medical profession: burns defined by, 16–21;
    history of, 131–47 passim; politics in, 192–
    93. *See also* caregivers
medications, use of, 73, 79–80
mental health. *See* burn patients, psychologi-
    cal status of
meshed skin, 156, *157*, 161, 181
Metamorphoses (Ovid), 38, 101, 102
metaphors: of burns, 30–31; of heat, 43
microstomia, 69
microwaved pie fillings, burns from, 43
Midsummer's eve, 100
Milliken, J. B., 160
mobility: recovery of, 181–82; restrictions
    on, 65–85 passim
Moncrief, J. A., 166
"Monster, The" (Crane), 12–13, 23, 34, 43,
    105
monsters, imagery of, 12–13
Moore, Francis D., 147, 154
mortality rate, from burns, 5, 142, 151, 155,
    166, 177–79
Morton, William, 140
motorcycle accidents, burns associated with,
    152–54
motorcycle exhaust pipes, burns from, 43
Moyer, Carl A., 142, 166
mummies, imagery of, 79, 103
mummification, 53
Munster, Andrew M., 190
Munster, Andrew, 44
muscle: atrophy of, 53–54; damage to, 18,
    53–54, 73
musculoskeletal system. *See* bone; muscle
myrrh, 133, 134
myths: about fire and burns, 89–104 passim;
    definition of, 89. ‹MDBR›See also specific
    groups

Nagasaki, destruction of, 39, 104
Nakazawa, Keiji, 124
napalm: burns from, 42, 61, 105–7, *106*;
    treatment of burns from, 39
National Burn Information Exchange
    (NBIE), 190
National Burn Victims Foundation, 195–96
National Fire Protection Association, 187
National Institutes of Health, 169
Native Americans: burn treatments of, 134;
    fire mythology of, 92, 94
natural gas explosions, 2, 29

Neesom, Liam, 115
Nelson, D. D., 188
Nero (Roman emperor), 61
nerves, damage to, 73
New Haven Rialto Theater fire, 145
New Orleans, fire in, 125
Nicholson, Jack, 113
Nietzsche, Friedrich, 91
Nightmare on Elm Street (film), 109, 113, 204. *See also* Freddy Krueger
Nines, Rule of, 18
Norse mythology, 99
novels, burn imagery in, 121–24
nuclear reactors, burns from, 42. *See also* radiation burns
nuclear weapons, fear of, 39
nurses, as caregivers, 28
Nusku, 91
nutrition, burn patients' need for, 53, 167–68
nutritionists, as caregivers, 28, 53, 168

occlusive dressings, 143
Occupational Safety and Health Administration (OSHA), U.S., 45
occupational therapists, as caregivers, 28, 53, 84, 171
O'Connor, N. E., 160
oil of turpentine, as burn treatment, 137. *See also* turpentine
oils. *See* carron oil; castor oil; cooking oil; elder-oil; linseed oil; olive oil
Oklahoma City: bombing in, 147; smoke alarm program in, 187
O'Leary, Hazel, 119
olive oil, as burn treatment, 133, 134
Ollier, Louis, 143
Ondaatje, Michael, 34
onions, as burn treatment, 135
open fires, burns from, 36, 44, 60
open-hearth steel production, burns from, 36
Orpheus, 102
Osiris, 102
Osler, William, 7
Ovid, 38, 101, 102
oxidation, 40, 205

Pachacamac, 92
Padgett, Earl Calvin, 143
pain: associated with burns, 17, 22; attempts to relieve, 73, 79–80; fear of, 31

pain-killers, use of, 73, 79–80
palmar fibrosis (Dupuytren's contracture), 138
Paracelsus, 156
Paré, Ambroise, 131, 135–36, 138
Parinder, Geoffrey, 92
Parkinson, Thomas, 138
Parkland formula, 154
partial thickness burns, definition of, 19
Passavant, G., 139
Pasteur, Louis, 164
patient controlled analgesia (PCA), 79
patients. *See* burn patients
pemphigus, burns from, 18
penicillin, 165
Persia: burn treatments in, 133; fire mythology of, 92
Peters, W. J., 156
Petro, Jane A., 80
petroleum products, burns from, 36, 131
Phaethon, imagery of, 37–38
Phantasma de la Opereta (film), 203
Phantom of Hollywood, The (film), 203
Phantom of the Opera, imagery of, 89, 108, 109, 110–13, *112*, 115, 201–4
Phantom of the Paradise (film), 203–4
Phoenix, Arizona, naming of, 103
phoenix, imagery of, 6–7, 89, 102–4, 185
Phoenix Society for Burn Survivors, Inc., 7, 103, 130, 187, 195
Phuc, Kim, 107
physical therapists, as caregivers, 28, 53, 84, 171, 181
physicians: as caregivers, 28; as decision-makers, 74–75
picric acid, as burn treatment, 144, 157
pig skin, grafting of, 156, 158
pinch grafts, 142, 143
Plague, The (Camus), 199
plasma, 154, 162
plastic surgery, 175, 180
Plato, 98
Please Let Me Die (film), 29, 69, 83
Pliny the Elder, 133
pneumonia, 50, 54
Pollock, G. D., 157
polymyxin cream, 166
Portland (Maine), fire in, 124–25
postmortem analysis, 178
post-traumatic stress syndrome (PTSS), 4, 32, 55, 172
"pourquoi" tales, 94

powders of acetate, as burn treatment, 143
prehistory, 90 91
pressure therapy, 69–73, *72*, 137, 172
Price, Vincent, 202, 203
Private Eyes (Kellerman), 122
Prometheus, 91, 94
Prontosil, 165
propane tanks, burns from explosion of, 1–4, 42
prosthetics, 180
pseudomonas, 165–66
psychiatrists, as caregivers, 28, 84
pulp fiction, 122
Pygmy mythology, 92
pyromania, 30–31, 63. *See also* arson
Pythagoras, 90

Queen of Outer Space, The (film), 202
Quetzalcoatl, 103

radiation (process), 205
radiation burns, 17, 118, 119
Ragnarok, 33, 39, 92
Rains, Claude, 201
Rancho Los Amigos Hospital (Downey, Calif.), 196
reconstructive surgery, 172, 180
recovery. *See* burn patients; burn survivors; burn treatments
Reddish, Patricia M., 55, 82
red giants, 39
reepithelialization, 142
Reeser, Mary, 121
resins, as burn treatments, 132–33
respiration, interruptions of, 42, 54
Reverdin, J. L., 142
Rheinwald, J. G., 160
Riddler, 118
Right Stuff, The (Wolfe), 32
risk assessment, 57
Roebuck, John, 139
Rome (ancient), burning of, 61
Romm, Sharon, 128
roofing tar, burns from, 42, 45
Rossi, Jean-Baptiste, 122
Rothenberg, David, 60
Rule of Nines, 18

Sacks, J. J., 188
Sacks, Oliver, 25
St. Luke's Regional Medical Center (Sioux City, Iowa), 194

saline baths, as burn treatment, 139, 143, 165
Salisbury, Roger, 171
salt (sodium chloride), as burn treatment, 142, 145, 154. *See also* saline baths
saltpeter, 134
Salzburg, C. A., 80
San Francisco, fires in, 125, 127
scald burns, 36, 44, 170, 188. *See also* boiling water; water, hot
Scarry, Elaine, 31
scar tissue, 69–73, 113, 172. *See also* contractures
Schindler's List (film), 61, 115
Schoeps, Margot, 14, 54
second-degree burns, 16, 18, 139
self-definition, fear of loss of, 33
Self-Help Source Book, The, 196
self-immolation, 62–63, 100, *107*, 107–8. *See also* suicide attempts, failed
Semmelweiss, Ignaz Phillip, 164
serum albumin, 154–55
shame, fear of, 32–33
Sharkey, P., 190
Sheffield, C. G., 174, 182
Shelley, Mary, 12
Shen Nung, 92
Shoma mythology, 92
Shriners, funding of burn centers by, 176, 189–90
Shriners Burn Institutes, 160, 176, 189–90
sickle cell disease, 54
sidewalks, burns from, 36
Sierra Leone mythology, 92, 95
Silvadene (R) cream, 166–67
silver nitrate (0.5 percent) solution, 166
silver sulfadiazine (Silvadene Cream), 52
Silvetti, A. N., 158
Simpson, James, 140
skin: debridement of, 29, 68–69, 75, 155; degrees (levels) of damage to, 18–19, 136, 138, 139; escharotomy of, 67, *68*; functions of, 51–52; harvesting and storage of, 159; as membrane between self and outer world, 11, 51–52; Stevens-Johnson syndrome of, 17–18; treatment of, 155–61. *See also* artificial skin; eschar; scar tissue; skin culturing
skin culturing, 155, 160–61
skin grafts: history of use of, 136, 142–43, 146, 155–56; long-term care of, 85, 181; types of, 155–56
slash-and-burn agriculture, 90

Slaughterhouse Five (Vonnegut), 61
Slavonic mythology, 92
Smith, Mary-Ann Tirone, 122
Smith-Meek, M., 190
smoke alarms, 187
smoke burns, 1
smoking, associated with burns, 121, 186, 188. *See also* cigarette (and cigar) burns
smoldering, 206
Sneve, H., 142, 145
Snitker, David, 22
social limitations, 74–79, 195–96
Social Security, 26, 169, 173
social workers, as caregivers, 28, 84
Socrates, 98
Sodom and Gomorrah, 96
Soelle, Dorothee, 55
Soma, 92, 93
Sorcerer's Apprentice, 102, 109
space heaters, burns from, 44
Speed (film), 110, 120
Spence, Basil, 103
Spiderman, 118
Spielberg, Steven, 61
spine boards, use of, 74
spirit of wine, as burn treatment, 139
spirituality, 83–84, 184
spontaneous human combustion, 40, 120–21
Stanford, Joseph, 122
staphylococcal infections, 134, 164, 165
steam, potential for burns from, 170
Stevens-Johnson syndrome, burns from, 17–18
stigma, 33
stigmata, 105
"stocking" burns, 60
streptococcal infections, 134, 164, 165
Stryker frames, 73
stump burning, 135
Subrahmanyam, M., 159
substance abuse, 55
suicide attempts, failed, 25, 62–63
Sulfamylon (R) cream, 166
sulfanilamide, 157, 165
sulfonamides, 165
sulfur, 134
sun, burns from, 39, 43. *See also* sunburn-type burns
sunburn-type burns, 2, 18, 19, 36
superficial burns, definition of, 19
super-heroes, 105, 118–19

Superman, imagery of, 118
support groups, 195
surgery, history of, 140
Surt, 92
survival, changing criteria for, 80. *See also* burn survivors
suttee, 61–62
Sutton, G., 194
sweatshop conditions, potential for burns in, 45, 188
synthetic skin, 155, 158–59
systemic antibiotics, 167

taboos about burns, 12
Tagliacozzi, Gaspare, 136, 138, 142
Tamayo, Rufino, 128
Tammuz, 102
Tampa Bay Regional Burn Unit, 198
Tampa General Hospital, 196
tangential excision, 156
Tanner, J. C., 156
tannic acid, as burn treatment, 143–44, 145–46, 157, 165
tanning salons, burns from, 43
Tarantula (film), 119
Tepplica, David, 130
Teutonic mythology, 92
Texas Chain Saw Massacre (film), 113
Them (film), 119
theriaca, 135
thermoregulation, 51
Thiersch, Carl, 143
thiosulfates, 136
third-degree burns, 16, 18
third-world countries, burns in, 44
Thompsonian school, 141
Threads (film), 39
Threefold Lotus Sutra, 63
Tibetan monks, burn treatments of, 134
Tin-Tan, 203
titanium dioxide, 157
Ton, Mary Ellen, 22
topical antibiotics, 167
Topley, E., 163
total body surface area (TBSA), 18
Towering Inferno (film), 119, 120
Tower of Babel, 94, 102
toxic epidermal necrosis syndrome (TENS), burns from, 18
transient organic mental syndrome, 55
translocation, of bacteria, 165
Trap for Cinderella (Rossi), 122

treatment, definition of, 15–16. *See also* burn
    treatments
tree saps, 132–33
trial by fire, 48
Triangle Shirtwaist fire, 45, 188
trickster, myths of, 94, 109
Turner, Alice, 98, 128
turpentine, as medical treatment, 137. *See
    also* oil of turpentine

unconsciousness, 75
Underhill, Frank, 145, 154
University of Michigan, 190
Ut, Huynh Cont ("Nick"), 61, 105–7, *106*

Vaseline, 157
Vedic mythology, 92–93, 100
Vietnam conflict, 39
vinegar, as burn treatment, 134
volcanic eruptions, burns from, 40
volcanic lava, burns from, 36, 43
Vonnegut, Kurt, 61

Wallace, A. F., 165
Ward, Vincent, 61
waterbed heating elements, burns from, 47
water heater pilot lights, burns from, 57
wax. *See* beeswax; hair removal wax

wax of oil (cerate), as burn treatment,
    139
Webber, Andrew Lloyd, 111, 115
Weidenfield, 142
Whose Life Is It Anyway? (play), 73
Wiley, Robert G., 196
Wily Coyote, 108
wine, as burn treatment, 133, 134, 165
Winslade, William, 80
Wiseman, Richard, 135, 137
witches, burning of, 97, 113
Wolfe, J. R., 143
Wolfe, Tom, 32
Woman's Face, A (film), 201
World Burn Congress, 187, 195
wounds: definition of, 17; inflicted during
    healing process, 29–30

xenografts (heterografts), 155, 156, 158
Xiuhecyhtli, 92

Young Men and Fire (Maclean), 40, 124
Yule logs, 100

Zabriskie Point (film), 120
Zawacki, Bruce, 80
zombies, imagery of, 79
Zoroastrianism, 92